£17.99

Milady's

HAIR-CARE
PRODUCT &
INGREDIENTS
DICTIONARY

JOHN HALAL

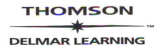

THOMSON

DELMAR LEARNING

Australia Canada Mexico Singapore Spain United Kingdom United States

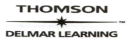

THOMSON

DELMAR LEARNING

Hair-Care Product & Ingredients Dictionary
John Halal

President, Milady:
Dawn Gerrain

Director of Production:
Wendy A. Troeger

Director of Marketing:
Donna Lewis

Director of Editorial:
Sherry Gomoll

Production Coordinator:
Nina Tucciarelli

Channel Manager:
Stephen Smith

Developmental Editor:
Judy Aubrey Roberts

Composition;
Type Shoppe II Productions

Editorial Assistant:
Courtney VanAuskas

Library of Congress Cataloging-in-Publication Data
Halal, John.
  Milady's hair care product ingredients dictionary/John Halal.
  p. cm. Includes bibliographical references.
  ISBN 1-56253-919-1
  1. Hair preparations—Dictionaries. 2. Hair—Care and hygiene. I. Title: Hair care product ingredients dictionary. II. Title.
  TT969.H35 2002
  646.7'24'0284—dc21
                2002031286

NOTICE TO THE READER

Publisher does not warrant or guarantee any of the products described herein or perform any independent analysis in connection with any of the product information contained herein. Publisher does not assume, and expressly disclaims, any obligation to obtain and include information other than that provided to it by the manufacturer.

The reader is expressly warned to consider and adopt all safety precautions that might be indicated by the activities herein and to avoid all potential hazards. By following the instructions contained herein, the reader willingly assumes all risks in connection with such instructions.

The Publisher makes no representation or warranties of any kind, including but not limited to, the warranties of fitness for particular purpose or merchantability, nor are any such representations implied with respect to the material set forth herein, and the publisher takes no responsibility with respect to such material. The publisher shall not be liable for any special, consequential, or exemplary damages resulting, in whole or part, from the readers' use of, or reliance upon, this material.

Contents

Preface

The average American woman uses 27 personal care beauty products each day, with an annual cost of about $350.00. In 2002, sales of hair care products in the United States increased by approximately 20 percent, to over 50 million dollars.

Advertising bombards us with an endless assortment of miracle creams and magic lotions that claim to make us look younger and more beautiful. Do these products really live up to their promises? Some cost more . . . much more. Are they worth the additional expense? Are they safe? How are we to know which products to buy?

Although most consumers are concerned about the effectiveness, safety, and value of the hair care products they buy and use, there is little reliable information available about those products. The overwhelming majority of information that consumers receive is paid for by the manufacturer and shouldn't be believed without scrutiny. If it seems too good to be true, it usually is.

Milady's Hair-Care Product & Ingredients Dictionary separates fact from fiction and helps you determine a product's effectiveness, safety, and value. The information in this book empowers consumers and salon professionals with an understanding of what is actually in those bottles and why it is there. If you have tried to read a product's list of ingredients but were intimidated by long unpronounceable words that seem to be written in some exotic, foreign language, this book is for you. With this book and a little practice, anyone can translate the ingredients "secretly" listed, in small print, on the back of the bottle. Those who don't understand the ingredient "language" are relegated to reading only the exaggerated marketing claims prominently listed, in big print, on the front of the bottle.

Milady's Hair-Care Product & Ingredients Dictionary contains accurate, reliable, and understandable definitions for the majority of ingredients currently being used in hair care products, including shampoos, conditioners, styling aids, permanent waves, haircoloring, chemical hair relaxers, chemical depilatories, and sunscreens. Although this dictionary does not specifically list skin care ingredients, skin and hair are similar in structure, and many hair care ingredients are also used in skin care.

Introductory chapters explain how to best use the dictionary. Section I explains how the Food, Drug, and Cosmetic Act, and the Fair Packaging and Labeling Act, affect the nomenclature and regulations that apply to product labeling. The distinction between drugs and cosmetics is clearly explained, along with how that distinction affects the use and labeling of ingredients. There is also an explanation of the Occupational Safety and Health Administration (OSHA) regulations that determine which ingredients are listed on Material Safety Data Sheets (MSDSs) and how they are listed.

Section II lists different ingredient functions. This section explains why the ingredient is being used. Each function contains an easy-to-understand explanation of that function, how it works, and the desired effect of the ingredient.

Section III contains a comprehensive alphabetical listing of the major ingredients likely to be found in hair care products. Definitions are listed by their International Nomenclature of Cosmetic Ingredients (INCI) name and include the phonetic pronunciation, common name and other names, plus the ingredient's primary function, its chemical class, and the type of product in which it is most likely to be found. Hazardous chemicals and those that are known to cause adverse reactions are also indicated.

And section IV contains a list of references and resources complete with mailing addresses, telephone numbers, and Web sites that make it easy to obtain additional information.

Dedication

This book is dedicated
to my mother, Alice,
the best mom in the world.

Acknowledgements

I would like to thank the following individuals who provided me with information and helped me with the research for this book.

Ken Klein
President
Cosmetech Laboratories, Inc.

Steve Hudson
Marianna, Inc.

I would also like to thank all the instructors and administrative staff at Honors Beauty College, Inc. for their assistance and patience.

Section I

Product Regulation and Ingredient Labels

The Federal Food, Drug, and Cosmetic Act, and the Regulation of Cosmetics

This dictionary is designed to help you evaluate the performance, safety, and value of the hair care products that you buy and use. All retail hair care products must contain a list of ingredients on the product label, but in order to understand those ingredients, we need to be aware of the government regulations that affect the product's classification, and the labeling and listing of those ingredients.

The primary regulations concerning cosmetics are included in the amended Federal Food, Drug, and Cosmetic Act (FDCA) of 1938, which controls all cosmetics made or distributed in interstate commerce, and specifically prohibits unsafe products and those that are not truthfully labeled. With the exception of color additives that are subject to premarket approval, enforcement of the FDCA must generally occur after the product is already on the market.

Retail cosmetics are also subject to the Fair Packaging and Labeling Act (FPLA) of 1966 and are required to contain a full list of ingredients on the product label. Professional cosmetic products, however, are exempt from the FPLA and are not required to list any ingredients. Professional products fall under the jurisdiction of the Occupational Safety and Health Administration (OSHA), which requires that the manufacturer provide a Material Safety Data Sheet (MSDS) that lists only the hazardous ingredients. Additional regulations for cosmetics are also authorized under the Consumer Product Safety Act, the Federal Anti-Tampering Act, and the Federal Trade Commission, which regulates cosmetic advertising.

The Distinction Between Drugs and Cosmetics

The distinction between over-the-counter (OTC) drugs and cosmetics is important because of the differences in the way they are manufactured, marketed, and labeled. As a general rule, drugs cause a physiological change in the body whereas cosmetics are limited to changes in appearance.

Since you will undoubtedly be reading the product ingredients from the label, you also need to know how the labels of drugs and cosmetics differ.

The FDCA defines cosmetics as:

1. Articles intended to be rubbed, poured, sprinkled, or sprayed on, introduced into, or otherwise applied to the human body or any part thereof for cleansing, beautifying, promoting attractiveness, or altering the appearance; and
2. Articles intended for use as a component of any such articles, except that such term shall not include soap.

Note that soap is not included and has been explicitly omitted from the definition of a cosmetic. For some reason, soaps that are used to clean the human body are not required to list any ingredients.

The FDCA defines drugs as:

B.   Articles intended for use in the diagnosis, cure, mitigation, treatment, or prevention of disease in man or other animals; and

C.   Articles (other than food) intended to affect the structure or any function of the body of man or other animals.

Contrary to what many think, the distinction between drugs and cosmetics is based on the intended use of the product, not its chemical composition. The intended use of a product is determined by the representations made for the product in its labeling; that is, from "any display of written, printed, or graphic matter" on the container, or on any materials that accompany the product.

The distinction between deodorants and antiperspirants is a perfect example. Deodorants are classified as cosmetics whereas antiperspirants are classified as drugs. Deodorants are intended to absorb perspiration or mask its odor. Deodorants are classified as cosmetics because they only claim to cover up or hide the odor caused by perspiration. Antiperspirants, on the other hand, are classified as drugs because they claim to retard or stop the perspiration that causes the odor. Cosmetics claim to cleanse, beautify, promote attractiveness, or alter the cosmetic appearance. Drugs claim to affect the structure or any function of the body.

Cosmetics include shampoos, conditioners, styling aids, permanent waves, chemical hair relaxers, chemical depilatories, hair dyes, bleaches, and rinses because these products claim to alter the appearance of the hair without affecting any function of the body. Although most shampoos are classified as cosmetics, antidandruff shampoos are classified as drugs because they are intended to cure, treat, or prevent a disease (dandruff).

Hair treatments that claim to make the hair appear thicker or fuller are classified as cosmetics, but products that claim to increase hair growth and make the hair grow thicker or fuller are classified as drugs. Although many hair products may claim to increase hair growth, Minoxidil (Rogaine) and Finasteride (Propecia) are the only two drugs approved by the Food and Drug Administration (FDA) for that purpose.

Many other products that are commonly thought of as cosmetics by the general public are, in fact, classified as over-the-counter drugs by the FDA. These products include fluoride and antiplaque toothpastes and mouthwashes. Sunscreens that list a sun protection factor (SPF) are intended to prevent sunburn and are therefore classified as drugs, while self-tanning products or those that claim to promote an even tan are classified as cosmetics.

Since cosmetics are subject to far fewer regulations than drugs, most manufacturers are pleased to be able to control a product's classification by merely describing the product within the intended uses outlined in the definition of cosmetics. But cosmetic and drug claims are not always mutually exclusive. A product intended for both cosmetic and drug use must comply with the regulations that govern both product classifications. One example would be a makeup foundation with a sunscreen that claims both sun protection and cosmetic benefits, an antidandruff shampoo that is also marketed to make the hair more manageable, or fluoride toothpaste that also claims to whiten teeth.

Recently, many within the industry have discussed the need to have a third category of products between drugs and cosmetics. Although the term "cosmeceutical" has been widely used to identify this proposed category, the FDA insists that there can be no new category under the FDCA, and that those products that make both drug and cosmetic claims must comply with both the drug and cosmetic regulations.

Product Identification

All cosmetics must contain an accurate statement of the net contents in English (fluid ounces) and metric (milliliters) units, and the name and address of the manufacturer, packer, or distributor, including the zip code. If the name that appears on the container is not the manufacturer, it must be prefaced by an explanatory phrase such as "Distributed by," "Manufactured for," or "Packaged by."

Declaration of Ingredients

An ingredient declaration must appear on the outermost retail container of all retail cosmetics. But since that requirement is limited to the sale of retail cosmetics, gifts, free samples, testers, and products sold to beauty salons solely for professional use are exempt from ingredient labeling and need not list any ingredients.

FDA regulations allow the use of three different formats for the ingredient declaration. The manufacturer is free to choose any of these three labeling methods and has no obligation to indicate which method was used.

Ingredients can be listed in order of predominance by weight or volume except that color additives may be grouped at the end of the list without regard to predominance, and ingredients in the product at 1 percent or less may be grouped at the end of the list without regard to predominance.

Although a fragrance must be declared, the ingredients used in the fragrance need not be listed. Fragrances may appear on the product listing simply as "fragrance."

Product Labeling of Over-the-Counter Drugs

In 1999, the FDA published regulations requiring nonprescription over-the-counter drugs, including cosmetic drugs, to carry labeling information in a uniform format and to separate that information from any other information such as cosmetic labeling. The additional information must be in the following order and enclosed in a box separated by black lines.

1. Title "Drug Facts"
2. Active ingredients including the amount in each dosage unit
3. Purpose of the product (for example, antidandruff shampoo)
4. Indications for use as permitted by the FDA
5. Any applicable warnings such as contraindications or possible side effects

The labeling must also declare all the inactive ingredients. Products marketed solely as OTC drugs must list the inactive ingredients in alphabetical order. Products marketed for cosmetic as well as drug use must list the inactive ingredients in order of predominance.

The Food and Drug Administration Modernization Act (FDAMA) of 1997 is the first major comprehensive reform of the FDCA since the 1960s. FDAMA requires that OTC drug labeling bear the amount or concentration of each active ingredient in the product as well as a full list of inactive ingredients. The FDAMA also eliminates what the FDA considers unsupported, absolute, or confusing terms such as "sunblock," "waterproof," "all day protection," and "visible and/or infrared light protection." Suntanning products that do not contain a sunscreen must also display a warning concerning the risk of sunburn.

Misbranded Cosmetics

According to the FDA, the term "misbranded" refers to statements, designs, or pictures used in product labeling that are explicitly "false or misleading" or that are misleading because the labeling omits a material fact about the product or the consequences of its use. The FDA has determined that cosmetics that use the terms "hair grower," "rejuvenating cream," "scalp food," "nourishing cream," "skin tonic," "wrinkle eradicator," or are represented as valuable because of their vitamin content are misbranded. Cosmetic products that contain vitamins may be considered misbranded if their labeling implies that the vitamins offer any kind of nutrient or health benefit.

Each cosmetic manufacturer is responsible for using only safe and suitable ingredients in its products, and for substantiating the safety of both the ingredients and the finished product. According to the FDA Labeling Handbook, "A cosmetic is considered misbranded if its safety has not adequately been substantiated, and it does not bear the following conspicuous statement: Warning: The safety of this product has not been determined."

Hair Dyes

Although the FDA must approve all color additives through regulation before they may be used in cosmetic products, "coal tar hair dye" colors are exempt as long as they comply with the specific regulations that apply to their use and labeling. The following warning statement must appear on the product containers:

> "Caution—This product contains ingredients which may cause skin irritation on certain individuals and a preliminary test according to the accompanying directions should first be made. This product must not be used for dyeing the eyelashes or eyebrows; to do so may cause blindness."

Self-Regulation

In recognition of its responsibility to provide safe cosmetic products and in order to avoid the need for additional mandatory controls by the FDA, the cosmetic industry has voluntarily chosen to fund private cosmetic ingredient safety reviews. The Research Institute for Fragrance Materials (RIFM), founded in 1966, has performed over 66,000 studies and acquired valuable information on more than 4,500 substances of interest to the cosmetic industry.

The Cosmetic Ingredient Review (CIR) was established in 1976 by the Cosmetic Toiletries and Fragrance Association (CTFA). Under the direction of the CIR, experts in the fields of dermatology, toxicology, and chemistry have reviewed over 800 ingredients and published reports in the *International Journal of Toxicology*. All CIR meetings are open to the public.

Hypoallergenic

There is a good deal of confusion concerning the meaning of the term "hypoallergenic." Cosmetics that claim to be hypoallergenic minimize the use of common allergens, but that does not guarantee that hypoallergenic products won't cause an allergic reaction in some individuals.

Antimicrobials

The FDA is currently reviewing the use of triclosan as an antimicrobial drug agent in body and hand-wash products, both in regard to its effectiveness and the role of antimicrobial products in the development of bacterial resistance. The FDA has suggested that antimicrobial soaps are no more effective than ordinary soaps at reducing bacteria on the skin surface. The FDA has warned manufacturers of antibacterial hand lotions that the dosage form (a lotion) and the claims (lasting antibacterial effect) are not included in proposed regulations for either antimicrobial first aid antiseptics or OTC health care antimicrobial wash products.

Section II

Product Ingredients

Ingredient Functions

Ingredients are listed in this section based on the function they perform in a finished hair care product. Many hair care ingredients have multiple functions and may be included in more than one category; therefore, the ingredients are listed according to their most common function. Some ingredients may have additional functions other than those listed here and may be used for reasons not described in this section.

Some ingredients may function as the active ingredients in OTC drugs. Although sunscreens and antidandruff shampoos are usually thought of as cosmetics, they are classified as OTC drugs by the FDA (see Section I).

Each function contains an explanation and description of the ingredients that serve that function. The functions are listed below.

Antidandruff
Antioxidants

Chelating Agents
Colorants
Conditioners — General
Conditioners — Moisturizers
Conditioners — Humectants
Conditioners — Antistatic
Depilatories
Fragrances
Hair Colorants
Hair Fixatives
Hair Waving and Straightening — Reducing Agents
Hair Straightening — Hydroxide Relaxers
Oxidizers
pH Adjusters
Preservatives
Propellants
Solvents
Sunscreens
Surfactants — General
Surfactants — Cleansing Agents
Surfactants — Emulsifying Agents
Surfactants — Foam Boosters
Thickeners

Antidandruff

Antidandruff agents are the active ingredients used in antidandruff products. In the United States, antidandruff products are defined as "a drug product used for the control of dandruff, seborrheic dermatitis, and psoriasis." Although Japan also regulates antidandruff products as drugs, in the European Union (EU) and other countries, antidandruff products are considered to be cosmetics and are controlled under cosmetic regulations, which may not require preclearance or premarket approval of active ingredients.

Each day, dead cells are shed from the skin's surface (epidermis) and replaced by new cells that grow from the skin's deeper layer (dermis). This natural process of skin regeneration takes place all over the body, including the scalp. It is important to distinguish between this natural shedding of dead skin cells and the medical condition called dandruff.

Most cases of common dandruff aren't dandruff at all, but simply dry skin. The combination of a dry climate with low humidity and the frequent use of the harsh cleansers found in most shampoos (see surfactants) aggravate dry skin and scalp conditions and make the symptoms worse. Dry desert climates and cold northern winters usually exacerbate dry skin and scalp. Dry skin should be treated with conditioning shampoos that contain mild cleansers and moisturizers.

Unlike dry skin, dandruff is believed to be caused by microorganisms, especially the yeast *Pityrosporum ovale*. Antidandruff agents are the active ingredients used in over-the-counter drug products for the control of dandruff, seborrheic dermatitis, and psoriasis. These ingredients have been proven safe and effective for that purpose, and may also have a cosmetic purpose.

Antioxidants

Antioxidants are used to stabilize hair care products by preventing or retarding the oxidation that would otherwise cause a product to turn rancid and spoil. Antioxidants prevent oxidation by neutralizing free radicals. Free radicals are "super" oxidizers that not only cause an oxidation reaction but also produce a new free radical in the process. Normal oxidation deactivates the oxidizer and stops the reaction from continuing, but the oxidation reaction caused by free radicals continues in a chain reaction that can go on forever. One free radical can oxidize millions of other compounds.

Antioxidants are free radical scavengers that stop the reaction from continuing. Antioxidants are ingredients used in cosmetics to prevent or retard a product from becoming rancid (the deterioration from a reaction with oxygen). They also play a vital role in maintaining the quality, integrity, and safety of cosmetic products. Typical cosmetic antioxidants include reducing agents and free radical scavengers.

Chelating Agents

Chelating agents, also called sequestrants, are ingredients that have the ability to combine with and deactivate metallic ions to eliminate unwanted reactions and stabilize the product. Chelating agents prevent the formation of metal precipitates, stabilize the product's color, and prevent oils from becoming rancid.

Soaps tend to leave a residue (soap scum) in hard water. Chelating agents are often added to soaps to improve performance by preventing the precipitation of the metals (calcium and magnesium) found in hard water. Chelating agents may be added to clarifying or detoxifying shampoos to aid in the removal of products that leave a coating or buildup on the hair.

Chelating agents also stabilize cosmetic products and prevent unwanted changes in their appearance. Calcium and magnesium ions are incompatible with a variety of cosmetic products and may cause a product to deteriorate over time. Chelation of ions, such as iron or copper, helps retard oxidative deterioration of finished products. Chelating agents are also used in clarifying shampoos to help retard or remove the buildup of metals caused by shampooing in hard water.

Colorants

Colorings in this classification are added to hair care products to impart color to the finished product. Colorings that are used to impart color to the hair are classified under hair colorants. Insoluble colors are usually known as pigments.

In the United States, the European Union Member States, and many other countries, colorants are subject to a wide range of regulatory restrictions. With few exceptions, the labeling names for colorants in the United States and the European Union may be different. In the United States, all colorants (with the exception of haircolors) must be preapproved (see Hair colorants).

The permanently listed colors that are exempt from FDA certification include carotene, disodium EDTA-copper, henna, henna extract, mica, titanium dioxide, zinc oxide, and caramel.

Conditioners—General

Hair conditioning ingredients perform a variety of different functions. They enhance the appearance and feel of the hair, increase body or volume, facilitate styling, improve gloss and shine, and improve the texture of hair that has been damaged by chemical services or heat and mechanical styling tools. The three main types of conditioning ingredients are *moisturizers*, *humectants*, and *antistatic*. Many hair conditioners perform more than one function and are listed under all the functions they perform.

Conditioners—Moisturizers.   Most moisturizers are oils or fatty materials that are designed to replace the natural oils that may have been removed by the surfactants that are used in many shampoos. Moisturizers act as lubricants to help hair and skin remain soft, smooth, and supple. Many moisturizers are occlusive materials that form a water-impermeable film that restricts the escape of water vapor from the uppermost layers of the skin. Moisturizers remain on the surface to reduce flaking, and to improve the appearance of dry hair and skin.

Conditioners—Humectants.   Humectants are hydroscopic materials that attract and retain moisture from the atmosphere. Humectants are used in hair care products to retard moisture loss from the product during use and prevent the product from drying out, even if it is left uncapped. The glycerin that is often added to toothpaste is a perfect example. The effectiveness of humectants depends to a large extent on the ambient relative humidity. Humectants may not perform well in extremely dry, arid climates.

Conditioners—Antistatic. Static electricity is caused by the repulsion of like electrical charges. Brushing and combing removes electrons from the hair and transfers them to the brush or comb. Static electricity is the result of these negative electrical charges. Static electricity is more noticeable on clean hair and in dry climates with little moisture.

Antistatic agents are ingredients that alter the electrical properties of the hair by reducing their tendency to acquire an electrical charge. Antistatic agents are used as processing aids in the manufacture of cosmetics and play an important role in the formulation of hair care products that prevent the condition commonly known as "flyaway hair."

Opposing electrical charges attract each other. Most antistatic agents are positively charged (cationic) and attach themselves to the surface of the hair by the process of adsorption. Cationic antistatic agents are substantive to the hair and skin, and also perform as conditioners. Antistatic agents such as quaternary ammonium compounds (Quats) are frequently used in leave-in, antistatic detanglers and conditioners.

Depilatories

Chemical depilatories are the active ingredients used in cosmetic products that are designed to remove unwanted, superfluous hair. These chemicals destroy the mechanical strength of hair so that it can be removed from the skin surface by mild scraping or rubbing. Depilatories are generally identical to hair-waving and straightening products, but are formulated at a significantly higher pH.

Chemical depilatories are different from mechanical epilating products like waxes or tapes, which are melted and applied to the skin with pressure, then quickly removed by stripping from the skin, pulling the hair out by its root or fracturing it.

Fragrances

The product label listing of "Fragrance" or Parfum" indicates any natural or synthetic substance used to impart an odor to a cosmetic product. According to the International Fragrance Association, fragrances are ingredients that impart, enhance, or blend the odor of a cosmetic product. Fragrances may be obtained from synthetic or natural sources by either chemical or physical processes. Fragrances include aroma chemicals, essential oils, natural extracts, distillates, isolates, and oleoresins.

Hair Colorants

Hair Colorants are materials that impart color to the hair. The two main categories of haircoloring products are *nonoxidation haircolors* and *oxidation haircolors.*

Nonoxidation Haircolors. These include temporary color rinses and traditional semipermanent haircolor. Nonoxidation haircolors are deposit-only haircolors that are not capable of lightening the natural hair color. They use preformed dyes with a high molecular weight that are unable to penetrate the hair shaft. Nonoxidation haircolors coat the outer portion of the hair without involving a chemical change in either the hair or the product. Their physical action produces a temporary change in hair color. The hair should return to its original color within one to eight shampoos, depending on the condition of the hair and the haircoloring product used.

Oxidation Haircolors. These include demipermanent haircolors (long-lasting semipermanent) and permanent haircolors. Oxidation haircolors involve a chemical change in both the hair and the product. They penetrate the hair and deposit small molecular weight colorless compounds that are oxidized into colored dyes inside the hair fiber. Oxidation haircolors are mixed with developer, usually hydrogen peroxide, immediately before use. The chemical action of oxidation haircolors produces a longer lasting color, with a permanent change in the natural hair color.

Demipermanent haircolors are also called deposit-only haircolors because they are designed to deposit color on the hair without changing or lightening the natural hair color. Deposit-only colors fade slowly with repeated shampoos.

Permanent haircolors are capable of depositing color and lightening the natural hair color in one process. Although the color deposited in the hair will fade slowly with repeated shampoos, the hair will not fade to its original natural color, but will eventually fade to the color to which it was lightened. In that regard, permanent haircolors are truly permanent.

Hair Fixatives

Hair fixatives are ingredients that impart hair-holding or style-retention properties to hair. Most hair fixatives used in styling lotions and hairsprays are polymers and gums that form a film on the surface of the hair. Substances that make the hair hydrophobic (repel water) are preferred because they retard the hair's tendency to absorb water and make it limp. Although some hair conditioning agents provide similar effects, this listing is limited to those film formers that are believed to be particularly suitable hair fixatives.

Hair Waving and Straightening—Reducing Agents

Hair waving and straightening agents (reducing agents) create a permanent change in the hair's wave pattern. These ingredients are thio compounds (mercaptans) that break disulfide bonds by a process called reduction. An oxidizing neutralizer, usually hydrogen peroxide, is used to rebuild the broken disulfide bonds after the hair has been placed in its new shape. This process is considered permanent because hair treated with reducing agents retains its new shape after shampooing.

Reducing agents do not actually curl hair; they simply soften it and allow it to conform to a new shape. Hair that is wrapped on rods conforms to the shape of the rod. The same reducing agents can also be used to straighten curly hair by stretching it straight instead of wrapping it on rods. The neutralizers used with reducing agents are oxidizers that permanently reform the hair fibers (disulfide bonds) in their new shape, either curly or straight.

Hair Straightening—Hydroxide Relaxers

Although reducing agents can be used to straighten curly hair, they may not be strong enough to effectively straighten coarse or extremely curly hair. Hydroxide relaxers are highly alkaline solutions that break disulfide bonds by a process called lanthionization, which is completely different from the reaction of the reducing agents used in hair waving and straightening.

After processing hair with a hydroxide relaxer, the relaxer is rinsed from the hair, and either a neutralizing shampoo or normalizing (neutralizing) lotion is applied. Hydroxide neutralizers are not the same as the oxidizing neutralizers used with reducing agents. Hydroxide neutralizers are acidic solutions that neutralize the remaining alkaline residues left behind by the relaxer. Although this process is more effective for extremely curly hair, hair that has been straightened with hydroxide relaxers cannot be permanently waved into a curly shape.

Oxidizers

Oxidizers are chemicals that contribute oxygen to another substance, causing that substance to become oxidized. Oxidizers are used as developers in haircolorants to form the synthetic dyes that add color to the hair. Oxidizers are used in higher concentrations in hair lighteners to destroy the natural pigment (melanin) and lighten natural hair color. Oxidizers are also used as neutralizers for hair waving and straightening (reducing agents).

pH Adjusters

pH adjusters are chemicals (acids, alkalis, and buffering agents) that are used to control the pH of finished cosmetic products. Acids are added to neutralize alkalis and lower the pH of the finished product. Alkalis (bases) are added to neutralize acids or raise the pH of the finished product. Buffers resist changes in pH and are used to stabilize the pH of the finished product.

Preservatives

Preservatives are ingredients that prevent or retard microbial growth and protect cosmetic products from spoiling. Most cosmetic products can support the growth of microorganisms and would spoil without the addition of preservatives. Adding preservatives prevents damage to the product that would otherwise be caused by these microorganisms, and also protects the product from inadvertent contamination by the consumer during use. Most finished products contain more than one preservative, which controls a wider variety of microorganisms and also causes a synergistic effect that increases their effectiveness.

Ingredients used to protect products from oxidative damage are listed as Antioxidants.

Propellants

Propellants are chemicals used in aerosol hairsprays to propel the hairspray out of the can. Aerosol hairsprays consist of a hair fixative dissolved in a fast-drying solvent that is propelled from the can by the pressurized gas propellant in the can. Aerosol hairsprays are easier to use than pump hairsprays and produce a drier spray with smaller droplets.

Although it has been 23 years (1979) since the federal government banned the propellants that were blamed for depletion of the ozone layer, aerosol hairsprays continue to raise fears of environmental calamity in the minds of most consumers. Aerosol hairsprays may be slightly more expensive, but they are no more damaging to the environment than pump hairsprays.

Solvents

Solvents are liquids used to dissolve other ingredients found in finished cosmetic products. Although water is the most common solvent found in hair care products, solvents other than water are used in hairsprays and nail lacquers. Specific solvents are also used to extract essential oils and dissolve the dyes in hair colorants.

Sunscreens

Sunscreens are the active ingredients used in over-the-counter sunscreen products. The FDA classifies sunscreen products, which list a sunscreen protection factor (SPF), as over-the-counter drugs. Sunscreens are active ingredients that absorb, reflect, or scatter radiation in the ultraviolet range at wavelengths from 290 to 400 nanometers.

Organic sunscreens like oxybenzone, avobenzone, and DEA methoxycinnamate are chemically active ingredients that absorb ultraviolet light. Inorganic sunscreens like titanium dioxide and zinc oxide physically reflect or scatter ultraviolet light. Although inorganic sunscreens are often referred to as nonchemical sunscreens because they physically block ultraviolet rays rather than absorbing them chemically, inorganic sunscreens are still chemicals. The use of inorganic sunscreens is growing because they eliminate the possibility of allergic reactions in those individuals who are sensitive to organic sunscreens.

Surfactants—General

The term surfactant is a contraction for surface-active agent. Oil and water don't normally mix because of surface tension. All surfactants work by acting on the surface of oil and water. Surfactants lower the surface tension, which causes the oil and water to mix.

Surfactants are often classified by their ionic charge. Anionic surfactants have a negative charge and are normally used in shampoos as the primary cleanser (detergent). Cationic surfactants have a positive charge and are most often used as conditioners. Cationic surfactants are listed under Conditioners—Antistatic. Cationic surfactants also have antimicrobial properties and may also be used as a preservative. Nonionic surfactants do not have an ionic charge. Most nonionic surfactants are used as conditioners and foam boosters. Amphoteric surfactants have both anionic and cationic charges that are influenced by pH. The cationic charges prevail at an acid pH and the anionic charges prevail at an alkaline pH. Amphoteric surfactants are often used in baby shampoos.

Although surfactants are used for many different reasons and some surfactants perform more than one function, the three main functions are *cleansing agents*, *emulsifying agents*, and *foam boosters*.

Surfactants—Cleansing Agents.

Anionic surfactants are the main active ingredients in all shampoos. All other ingredients are added to improve the action of the surfactants or to alter the product's texture, color, fragrance, or feel. Although a single primary surfactant is usually responsible for cleansing the hair and scalp, other surfactants are often added to improve cleansing, reduce irritation, increase foam, and condition the hair.

The surfactants used in shampoos as cleansing agents have the ability to wet hair and skin, and remove, emulsify, and suspend dirt and oil so that it can be carried away with the rinse water. Although many cleansing agents produce foam, foam is not responsible for the cleansing properties of surfactants. Other surfactants are usually added to perform that function (see Foam Boosters).

The most common primary surfactants used in shampoos are 1) lauryl sulfates and 2) lauryl ether sulfates.

1) Lauryl sulfates (lauryl sulfate) are often used as the primary surfactant because they are inexpensive and are very good cleansers, but they can be damaging to the hair and irritating to the skin. Some of the most common examples include sodium lauryl sulfate, ammonium lauryl sulfate, and TEA lauryl sulfate.

2) Lauryl ether sulfates (laureth sulfate) are ethoxylated to produce a surfactant that is milder and less irritating. Some of the most common examples include sodium laureth sulfate, ammonium laureth sulfate, and TEA laureth sulfate. The degree of ethoxylation is determined by the amount of ethylene oxide that is added. An ethoxylation value of about three is usually preferred for cleansing ability and relative mildness. Higher ethoxylated lauryl sulfates—sodium lauroamphoacetate, alkylglucosides, and alkylglutamates—are surfactants that are often used to add mildness.

Surfactants—Emulsifying Agents.   Emulsifying agents are used to prepare emulsions, which is the core technology of most hair care products. The overwhelming majority of hair care products are emulsions. Emulsions are usually made from a blend of oils and water, and range in form from milks to creams with applications that are as varied as the processes that produce them.

The primary purpose of an emulsifying agent is to create a stable uniform product that ensures the quality of the product for at least three years during shipping, storage, distribution, and use. Emulsifiers provide the product's texture and thickness, and also contribute to its overall safety and effectiveness.

The ability of a surfactant to disperse and stabilize the emulsion also alters the feel of a product. When used properly, emulsifiers cause a product to liquefy and spread evenly when applied. When used improperly, emulsifiers cause a product to feel heavy and drag when applied, or create an undesirable sticky or tacky after-feel.

Emulsifiers also have the ability to disturb essential oils on the skin. The same emulsifiers that are used to attract and hold oils in the emulsion may also emulsify the essential lipids (oils) in the skin. Strong surfactants such as sodium lauryl sulfate and even milder emulsifiers can disturb the lipid-barrier properties of the skin. Emulsifiers may also increase irritation indirectly by damaging the barrier of the skin, which enhances absorption of other irritating materials such as preservatives, salts, or other active ingredients.

Surfactants—Foam Boosters.   Foam boosters are responsible for the rich, thick, creamy foam found in shaving soaps, shampoos, bubble baths, liquid soaps, mousses, and aerosol-dispensed foams. Foam boosters are cosurfactants that allow the surfactant molecules to pack better, which strengthen the foam and boost the foaming power. The most common cosurfactants are cocamide MEA, cocamide DEA, cocamidopropyl betaine, and other betaines.

Although foam is not responsible for the cleansing properties of shampoo, most shampoos are designed to produce dense foam because the consumer relates thick, rich foam with a quality shampoo. Foam has become an important aspect of shampoos. Shampoo should quickly produce a rich, dense, "flash foam" in the first stages of the shampooing process. The foam should remain during the process, even in the presence of sebum or oily conditioners, but should also rinse easily during the final stages.

Even without foam boosters, some foam is always generated by excess surfactant, and is an indication that sufficient shampoo is present to suspend all the dirt and oil. Foam also has a lubricating quality that allows the hands to move easily through wet hair, which aids in the mechanical removal of the emulsified dirt and oil.

A mild shampoo should gently cleanse the hair and scalp without causing irritation, dryness, or damage. Unfortunately, the surfactants that provide the best foam also exhibit the highest skin irritation. Although most mild surfactants such as ammonium lauryl ether sulfate do not irritate the skin, they are weak cleansers that produce a poor lather. Most formulators attempt to balance cleansing ability, lathering, and mildness, but mildness is often only obtained at the expense of effective cleansing and lathering. Most shampoos blend mild surfactants with surfactants that cleanse well and lather profusely.

Thickeners

Thickeners are ingredients that are used to increase the viscosity (thickness) of hair care products such as shampoos, conditioners, styling gels, and various other emulsions.

Gels are usually semisolids, and are clear to translucent. The viscosity ranges from a thickened, pourable liquid gel to a soft, solid stick. Gels can be thickened with synthetic polymers such as acrylic, vinyl, and alkylene/alkylene oxide, or natural polymers such as polysaccharides from plant or microbial origin that have been chemically modified. Improper use of thickeners can create a product that flakes, doesn't spread well, or leaves a sticky feel.

Section III

Alphabetical Listing of Hair Care Product Ingredients

Section III contains an alphabetical listing of ingredients commonly found in hair care products. Ingredients are listed according to their International Nomenclature of Cosmetic Ingredients (INCI) name and their common name with cross-references, when applicable. INCI names have ben adopted by the Cosmetic, Toiletry, and Fragrance Association and are approved by the FDA. INCI names are most likely to be the ones listed on the label of retail products and MSDS of professional salon products.

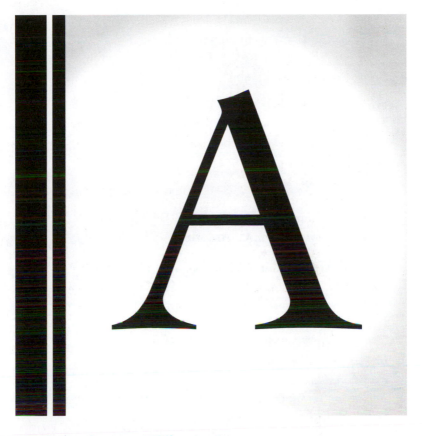

Abietic Acid (ab-ee-ET-ik AS-ud)

Definition: Abietic acid is an organic acid derived from wood rosin in the form of a slightly yellow crystalline powder.

Class: Carboxylic Acids

Function: Surfactant, Emulsifying Agent

Found in: Shampoos, Conditioners

Other Names: Sylvic Acid

Acacia (Uh-KAY-shuh)

Definition: Acacia is the dried, gummy material from the stems and branches of the African acacia tree *Acacia senegal.* It contains the complex polysaccharide called arabic acid and is used as a thickener.

A

Class: Natural ingredients, Gums, Thickeners
Function: Thickeners, Fixatives
Found in: Shampoos, Soaps, Conditioners, Styling Aids
Other Names: Gum Arabic

Acerola (ah-SER-oh-la)

Definition: Acerola is a natural source of ascorbic acid (vitamin C) obtained from the fruit of the West Indian cherry, *Malpighia punicifolia*.
Class: Natural Acid
Function: pH Adjuster
Found in: Shampoos, Conditioners, Styling Aids
Other Names: Vitamin C, Ascorbic Acid

Acetamide MEA (as-et-AM-eyed)

Definition: Acetamide MEA is a conditioner that is added to shampoos to improve wet combing and manageability. It also reduces the irritation caused by other surfactants that may be used as the primary cleanser.
Class: Alkanolamides
Function: Conditioner, Humectant, Foam Booster, Surfactant
Found in: Shampoos, Conditioners, Moisturizers
Other Names: N-acetyl ethanolamide, acetic acid monoethanolamide, Acetylcolamin

Acetamidopropyl Trimonium Chloride (as-et-AM-eyed-oh-pro-pil try-MO-nee-um KLOR-eyed)

Definition: Acetamidopropyl trimonium chloride is a quaternary ammonium compound used in shampoos and conditioners as an antistatic conditioner to prevent flyaway hair.
Class: Quaternary Ammonium Compounds
Function: Conditioners — Antistatic
Found in: Hair Conditioners, Bath Soaps and Detergents, Shampoos
Other Names: 3-N-N-N-Trimethyl-1-Propanamonium Chloride

A

Acetic Acid (uh-SEET-ik AS-ud)

Definition: Acetic acid is a carboxylic acid that is produced by the distillation of wood or the oxidation of alcohol by fermentation. Vinegar is a diluted and impure form of acetic acid produced by fermentation. Acetic acid is used to lower the pH.

Class: Carboxylic Acid

Function: pH Adjuster—Acid

Found in: Hair Colorants, Conditioners

Other Names: Ethanoic Acid, Ethylic Acid, Glacial Acetic Acid, Methanecarboxylic Acid

1-Acetoxy-2-Methylnaphthalene (ONE AS-et-oxy TOO METH-ul-nap-tha-leen)

Definition: 1-Acetoxy-2-Methylnaphthalene is an organic hair colorant that requires a patch test prior to use.

Class: Hair Colorants

Function: Hair Colorant

Found in: Hair Dyes, Hair Colorants

Other Names: 2-methyl-1-Naphthyl Acetate

Acetylated Lanolin (uh-SEET-ul-ayt-ed LAN-ul-un)

Definition: Acetylated lanolin is a nontacky, water-insoluble derivative of lanolin.

Class: Lanolin, Lanolin Derivatives

Function: Conditioner, Moisturizer

Found in: Conditioners—Moisturizer

Other Names: Hard Lanolin Acetate, Lanolin Acetate

Acid Black 1 (AS-ud BLAK)

Definition: Acid black 1 is an organic colorant.

Class: Diazo Color

Function: Colorant

Found in: Shampoos

Other Names: Acidal Black 10B, Amido Black 10B, Amino Black 10B

A

Acid Blue 9 (AS-ud BLOO)
Definition: Acid blue 9 is a triphenylmethane color.
Class: Colorants
Function: Colorant
Found in: Shampoos, Conditioners, Hair Colorants
Other Names: Blue No. 1, Brilliant Blue FCF

Acid Brown 13 (AS-ud BROUN)
Definition: Acid Brown 13 is a nitro color.
Class: Hair Colorant
Function: Hair Colorant
Found in: Hair Dyes, Hair Colorants
Other Names: Benzenesulfonic Acid

Acid Green 25 (AS-ud GREEN)
Definition: Acid green 25 is an anthraquinone color.
Class: Colorants
Function: Colorant
Found in: Shampoos, Conditioners
Other Names: Acid Green Anthraquinone, Green No. 201,
    m-toluenesulfonic acid

Acid Orange 3 (AS-ud OR-inj)
Definition: Acid orange is a nitro color.
Class: Colorants
Function: Hair Colorant
Found in: Hair Dyes, Hair Colorants
Other Names: Acid Yellow E, Amido Yellow E

Acid Red 14 (AS-ud RED)
Definition: Acid red 14 is a monoazo color.
Class: Colorants
Function: Hair Colorant
Found in: Hair Dyes, Hair Colorants
Other Names: Acide Rubine, Azo Rubin, Carmoisine

Acid Yellow 1 (AS-ud YEL-oh)
Definition: Acid yellow 1 is a nitro color.

A

Class: Colorants
Function: Hair Colorant
Found in: Hair Bleaches
Other Names: Citronin A, Flavianic Acid Sodium Salt,
   Yellow 403

Acrylate/Acrylamide Copolymer (uh-KRIL-ayts/uh-KRIL-am-eyed ko-PAHL-uh-mer)

Definition: Acrylate/acrylamide copolymer is a copolymer of
   acrylamide and acrylic acid, or methacrylic acid.
Class: Synthetic Polymers
Function: Hair Fixative
Found in: Styling Aids, Hairsprays
Other Names: Acrylamide-Acrylate Copolymer

Acrylate/Ammonium Methacrylate Copolymer (uh-KRIL-ayt/uh-MOH-nee-um meth-ah-KRIL-ayt ko-PAHL-uh-mer)

Definition: Acrylate/ammonium methacrylate copolymer is a
   polymer of ammonium methacrylate and acrylic acid, or
   methacrylic acid.
Class: Synthetic Polymer
Function: Hair Fixative
Found in: Styling Aids, Hairsprays
Other Names: Acrylate/Ammonium Methacrylate Copolymer

Acrylates Copolymer (uh-KRIL-ayts ko-PAHL-uh-mer)

Definition: Acrylates coplymer is a copolymer of two or more
   monomers of acrylic acid, or methacrylic acid.
Class: Synthetic Polymers
Function: Hair Fixative
Found in: Styling Aids, Hairsprays
Other Names: Acrylic/Acrylates Copolymer

Adipic Acid (ay-DIP-ik AS-ud)

Definition: Used as a flavor in foods and an acidifying agent
   in cosmetics. Occurs naturally in beets, but is commercially prepared in large quantities from natural gas or oil.

Class: Carboxylic Acid
Function: pH Adjuster
Found in: Permanent Waves
Other Names: Hexanedioic Acid, 1,4-Butanedicarboxylic
Acid

Alanine (AL-uh-neen)

Definition: A naturally occurring amino acid obtained from
the hydrolysis (degradation) of proteins. Used for market-
ing as a natural ingredient.
Class: Amino Acids
Function: Conditioner
Found in: Shampoos, Conditioners
Other Names: 2-Aminopropanoic Acid

Alcohol (AL-kuh-hawl)

Definition: Alcohol is ethyl alcohol that has not been dena-
tured. It is used as a solvent, bactericide, and astringent. It
does have a drying action on the skin and will sting the
eye.
Class: Alcohols
Function: Solvent, Bactericide, Astringent
Found in: Hair Dyes, Hair Colorants, Shampoos, Condition-
ers, Styling Aids, Hairsprays
Other Names: Ethanol, Undenatured, Ethyl Alcohol,
Undenatured

Alcohol Denatured (AL-kuh-hawl dee-NAY-churd)

Definition: Alcohol denatured is ethyl alcohol that is dena-
tured in accordance with the regulations of the U.S. Bu-
reau of Alcohol, Tobacco, and Firearms.
Class: Alcohols
Function: Solvent, Bactericide, Astringent
Found in: Hair Dyes, Hair Colorants, Shampoos, Condition-
ers, Styling Aids, Hairsprays
Other Names: Denatured Alcohol

A

Algin (AL-jin)

Definition: Algin is a polysaccharide extracted from the brown seaweed *Phaeophyceae* that is used to thicken and stabilize emulsions. Algin is present in the form of mixed salts that are extracted with the help of alkalis. Algin contains polymers of mannuronic and guluronic acids.

Class: Gum

Function: Thickener, Stabilizer

Found in: Conditioners

Other Names: Alginic Acid, Sodium Alginate, Sodium Polymannuronate

Allantoin (eh-LAN-tow-in)

Definition: Allantoin has been used medicinally for hundreds of years. It occurs naturally in comfey root and also in the excrement of maggots. Allantoin is commercially prepared by the oxidation of uric acid.

Class: Heterocyclic Compounds

Function: Conditioner

Found in: Shampoos, Conditioners

Other Names: Glyoxyldiuride, 3-Ureidohydantoin, Imidazolidinyl Urea

Aloe (AL-oh)

Definition: Aloe is any of the materials derived from the aloe plant, and includes gel, juice, powder, and extract.

Class: Biological

Function: Conditioner—Humectant

Found in: Shampoos, Conditioners, Styling Aids, Miscellaneous

Other Names: Aloe Vera, *Aloe andongensis* Extract, *Aloe barbadensis*

Aluminum Stearate (a-LOO-muh-num STEE-uh-rayt)

Definition: Aluminum stearate is the aluminum salt of stearic acid.

Class: Colorants
Function: Colorant, Thickener
Found in: Shampoos, Conditioners, Miscellaneous
Other Names: Aluminum Dihydroxide Stearate, Octadecanoic Acid

6-Amino-m-Cresol (uh-MEE-noh KREE-sol)

Definition: 6-Amino-m-Cresol is an aromatic amine hair colorant. Caution statements and a patch test are required.
Class: Amines, Phenols
Function: Hair Colorant
Found in: Hair Dyes, Hair Colorants
Other Names: 4-amino-3-hydroxytoluene, 6-amino-3-methylphenol

Aminomethyl Propanol (uh-MEE-no-METH-ul PRO-pen-ol)

Definition: Aminomethyl propanol (AMP) is an aliphatic alcohol that is widely used as an ammonia substitute to increase pH.
Class: Alkanolamines
Function: pH Adjuster
Found in: Hair Colorants, Permanent Waves, Hair Straighteners
Other Names: AMP, Aminoisobutanol, Isobutanolamine

4-Amino-2-Nitrophenol (uh-MEE-noh ny-troh FEE nol)

Definition: 4-amino-2-nitrophenol is an aromatic phenol hair colorant.
Class: Amines, Phenols
Function: Hair Colorant
Found in: Hair Dyes, Hair Colorants
Other Names: Amino hydroxynitrobenzene

m-Aminophenol (uh-MEE-noh-fee-nol)

Definition: m-Aminophenol is an aromatic amine hair colorant. Caution statements and a patch test are required.
Class: Amines, Phenols
Function: Hair Colorant

Found in: Hair Dyes, Hair Colorants
Other Names: Hydroxyaminobenzene, Hydroxyphenylamine

Ammonium Benzoate (uh-MOH-nee-um BEN-zoe-ayt)

Definition: Ammonium benzoate is the ammonium salt of benzoic acid.
Class: Organic Salts
Function: Preservative
Found in: Aerosol Hairsprays
Other Names: Benzoic Acid, Ammonium Salt

Ammonium Bicarbonate (uh-MOH-nee-um by-CAR-bun-ayt)

Definition: Ammonium bicarbonate is an inorganic salt that is used to adjust the pH of permanent waves.
Class: Inorganic Salt
Function: pH Adjusters
Found in: Permanent Waves
Other Names: Carbonic Acid, Monoammonium Salt

Ammonium Bisulfite (uh-MOH-nee-um by-SUL-fyt)

Definition: Ammonium bisulfite is an inorganic salt that is used in permanent waving and straightening.
Class: Inorganic Salt
Function: Hair Waving or Straightening—Reducing Agent
Found in: Permanent Waves, Styling Lotions
Other Names: Sulfurous Acid, Monoammonium Salt

Ammonium C12-15 Alkyl Sulfate (uh-MOH-nee-um al kul SUL-fayt)

Definition: Ammonium C12-15 alkyl sulfate is the ammonium salt of the sulfate of C12-15 alcohols. This is a common surfactant used in a wide variety of products.
Class: Alkyl Sulfate
Function: Surfactant—Cleansing Agent
Found in: Shampoos, Conditioners
Other Names: Ammonium C12-15 Alcohol Sulfate

A

Ammonium Chloride (uh-MOH-nee-um KLOR-eyed)

Definition: Ammonium chloride is an inorganic salt that is used to thicken products.

Class: Inorganic Salts

Function: Thickener

Found in: Shampoos, Permanent Waves, Bleaches, Miscellaneous

Other Names: Ammonium Muriate, Salmiac, Sal Ammoniac

Ammonium Cocoyl Isethionate (uh-MOH-nee-um KO-koyl eye-SETH-ee-oh-nayt)

Definition: Ammonium cocoyl isethionate is the ammonium salt of the isethionic acid found in coconuts.

Class: Isethionates

Function: Surfactant—Cleansing Agent

Found in: Shampoos, Conditioners

Other Names: Ammonium N-Cocoyl Isethionate

Ammonium Hydroxide (uh-MOH-nee-um hy-DRAHKS-yd)

Definition: Ammonium hydroxide is an inorganic alkali used to raise the pH.

Class: Inorganic Alkali

Function: pH Adjuster

Found in: Hair Dyes, Hair Colorants, Permanent Waves, Hair Straighteners, Bleaches

Other Names: Ammonia Solution, Ammonia Water

Ammonium Laureth Sulfate (uh-MOH-nee-um LOR-eth SUL-fayt)

Definition: Ammonium laureth sulfate is the ammonium salt of ethoxylated lauryl sulfate. Ethoxylated surfactants (ammonium laureth sulfate) are generally milder and less irritating to the skin than their nonethoxylated counterparts (ammonium lauryl sulfate). Ammonium laureth sulfate is commonly used as the primary cleansing agent in shampoos because it is inexpensive and provides rich,

A

abundant foam, even in hard water. It is an excellent cleanser that leaves the hair feeling very clean. Ammonium laureth sulfate is also more stable in acid-balanced shampoos than sodium laureth sulfate or TEA laureth sulfate.

Class: Alkyl Ether Sulfates, Ethoxylated Surfactants
Function: Surfactant—Cleansing Agent
Found in: Shampoos, Miscellaneous
Other Names: Ammonium Lauryl Ether Sulfate

Ammonium Lauroyl Sarcosinate (uh-MOH-nee-um LOR-oyl sar-KOHS-in-ayt)

Definition: Ammonium lauroyl sarcosinate is the ammonium salt of lauroyl sarcosine. Sarcosinates are mild foaming and cleansing agents. They are used in shampoos as secondary surfactants to improve the mildness, conditioning properties, and foaming power of other surfactants.

Class: Sarcosinates
Function: Surfactant—Cleansing Agent, Conditioner
Found in: Shampoos, Conditioners
Other Names: N-Lauroylsarcosine Ammonium Salt

Ammonium Lauryl Sulfate (uh-MOH-nee-um LOR-ul SUL-fayt)

Definition: Ammonium lauryl sulfate is the ammonium salt of lauryl sulfate. Ammonium lauryl sulfate is commonly used as the primary cleansing agent in shampoos because it is inexpensive and provides rich, abundant foam, even in hard water. It is an excellent cleanser that leaves the hair feeling very clean. Ammonium lauryl sulfate is more stable in acid-balanced shampoos than sodium lauryl sulfate or TEA lauryl sulfate. Ammonium lauryl sulfate is generally not as mild and is more irritating to the skin than the ethoxylated surfactant ammonium laureth sulfate.

Class: Alkyl Sulfates
Function: Surfactant—Cleansing Agent

Found in: Shampoos, Conditioners, Miscellaneous
Other Names: Dodecyl Ammonium Sulfate

Ammonium Myreth Sulfate (uh-MOH-nee-um MYR-eth SUL-fayt)

Definition: Ammonium myreth sulfate is the ammonium salt of ethoxylated myristyl sulfate. It is a mild foaming and cleansing agent and is slightly milder to the skin than sodium myreth sulfate.
Class: Alkyl Ether Sulfates
Function: Surfactant—Cleansing Agent
Found in: Shampoos, Conditioners
Other Names: Polyethylene Oxide Monotetradecyl Ether Sulfate Ammonium Salt

Ammonium Persulfate (uh-MOH-nee-um pur-SUL-fayt)

Definition: Ammonium persulfate is an inorganic salt that is used in powdered bleaches as a hair-lightening agent. Because it is known to cause scalp irritation, it is usually recommended for highlighting applications off the scalp.
Class: Inorganic Salts
Function: Oxidizer
Found in: Hair Bleaches, Highlighting Kits
Other Names: Diammonium Persulfate, Ammonium Peroxydisulfate

Ammonium Sulfite (uh-MOH-nee-um SUL-fyt)

Definition: Ammonium sulfite is an inorganic salt that is used in permanent waves and hair straighteners.
Class: Inorganic Salts
Function: Hair Waving and Straightening—Reducing Agent
Found in: Permanent Waves, Hair Straighteners
Other Names: Diammonium Sulfite, Diammonium Sulfonate

Ammonium Thioglycolate (uh-MOH-nee-um thy-oh-GLY-kuh-layt)

Definition: Ammonium thioglycolate is the ammonium salt of thioglycolic acid. Ammonia is added to thioglycolic acid as an alkalizing agent.

Class: Organic Salts, Thio Compounds

Function: Hair Waving and Straightening—Reducing Agents

Found in: Permanent Waves, Hair Straighteners

Other Names: Ammonium Mercaptoacetate

Amodimethicone (uh-moh-dy-METH-ih-kohn)

Definition: Amodimethicone is a silicone polymer used as a conditioner. It improves wet combing and adds shine without buildup.

Class: Siloxanes

Function: Conditioner—Moisturizer

Found in: Conditioners, Styling Lotions, Hairsprays, Hair Dyes, Hair Colorants

Other Names: Aminoethylaminopropylsiloxane Dimethylsiloxane Copolymer

Ascorbyl Palmitate (ah-SKOR-bil PAL-muh-tayt)

Definition: Ascorbyl palmitate is the ester of ascorbic acid and palmitic acid. It is used as an antioxidant and a fragrance ingredient.

Class: Esters, Polyols

Function: Antioxidant, Fragrance

Found in: Shampoos, Conditioners, Styling Aids, Miscellaneous

Other Names: Ascorbic Acid Palmitate, Palmitoyl L-Ascorbic Acid

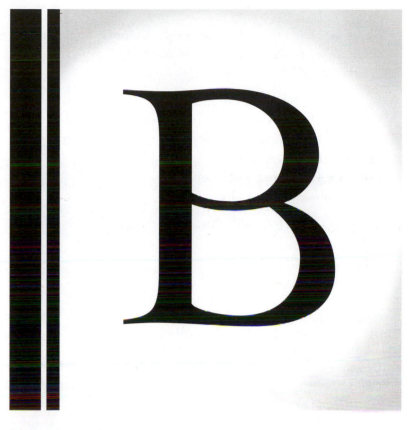

Basic Blue 9 (BAYS-ik BLOO)

Definition: Basic blue 9 is a thiazine color used as a hair colorant.

Class: Color Additives—Hair

Function: Hair Colorant

Found in: Hair Dyes, Hair Colorants

Other Names: Methylene Blue, Methylenium Ceruleum, Methylthionine Chloride, Solvent Blue

Basic Brown 17 (BAYS-ik BROUN)

Definition: Basic brown 17 is a monoazo color used as a hair colorant.

Class: Color Additives—Hair

B

Function: Hair Colorant
Found in: Hair Dyes, Hair Colorants, Coloring Shampoos
Other Names: 2-Naphthaleneaminium 8 Hydroxy-N,N,N-Trimethyl-Chloride

Basic Green 1 (BAYS-ik GREEN)

Definition: Basic Green 1 is a triphenylmethane color.
Class: Color Additives—Hair
Function: Hair Colorant
Found in: Hair Dyes, Hair Colorants
Other Names: Brilliant Green

Basic Orange 31 (BAYS-ik OR-enj)

Definition: Basic orange 31 is a hair colorant.
Class: Color Additives—Hair
Function: Hair Colorant
Found in: Hair Dyes, Hair Colorants
Other Names: CL Basic Orange 31

Basic Red 1 (BAYS-ik RED)

Definition: Basic red 1 is a xanthene colorant.
Class: Color Additives—Hair
Function: Hair Colorant
Found in: Hair Dyes, Hair Colorants
Other Names: CL 45160, Xanthium, 9-3, 6-Bis Dimethyl Chloride

Basic Violet 10 (BAYS-ik VY-uh-let)

Definition: Basic violet 10 is a xanthene colorant.
Class: Color Additive—Miscellaneous
Function: Hair Colorant
Found in: Hair Dyes, Hair Colorants
Other Names: Red No. 213, Rhodamine B

Basic Yellow 57 (BAYS-ik YEL-oh)

Definition: Basic yellow 57 is a monoazo hair colorant.
Class: Color Additive—Hair

Function: Hair Colorant
Found in: Hair Dyes, Hair Colorants
Other Names: 3-N,N,N-Trimethyl Benzenaminium
Chloride

Beeswax (BEEZ-waks)

Definition: Beeswax is the purified wax from the honeycomb
of the bee, *Apis mellifera*. It is commonly called white wax
when bleached and yellow wax when not bleached.
Class: Waxes
Function: Surfactant — Emulsifying Agent, Thickener
Found in: Shampoos, Conditioners, Styling Aids,
Miscellaneous
Other Names: Cera Alba, White Wax, Yellow Wax

Beetroot Red (BEET-root RED)

Definition: Beetroot red is a color additive that contains beta-
nine and is obtained from the roots of red beets.
Class: Color Additives
Function: Colorant
Found in: Shampoos, Conditioners, Styling Aids, Miscellaneous
Other Names: Betanine

Behanalkonium Chloride (beh-an-al-KOH-nee-um KHLOR-eyed)

Definition: Behanalkonium chloride is a quaternary ammo-
nium salt.
Class: Quaternary Ammonium Compounds
Function: Conditioners — Antistatic
Found in: Hair Conditioners, Leave-in Conditioners
Other Names: Ammonium Benzyldocoslyldimethyl Chloride,
Benzyl Docosyl Dimethyl Ammonium Chloride

Behenamide DEA (beh-an-AM-eyed)

Definition: Behenamide DEA is a mixture of ethanolamides
of behenic acid.
Class: Alkanolamides

B

Function: Conditioner, Surfactants — Foam Booster, Thickener
Found in: Shampoos, Conditioners, Miscellaneous
Other Names: Behenic Acid Diethanolamide, Diethanolamine Behenic Acid Amide

Beheneth-5 (BEH-en-eth)

Definition: Beheneth-5 is the polyethylene glycol ether of behenyl alcohol.
Class: Alkoxylated Alcohols
Function: Surfactants — Emulsifying Agent
Found in: Shampoos, Conditioners, Miscellaneous
Other Names: PEG-5 Behnyl Ether, Polyethylene Glycol Behenyl Ether

Behenyl Alcohol (BEH-en-ul AL-kuh-hawl)

Definition: Behenyl alcohol is a mixture of fatty alcohols consisting chiefly of n-docosanol.
Class: Fatty Alcohols
Function: Surfactants — Emulsifying Agent, Thickener
Found in: Shampoos, Conditioners, Miscellaneous
Other Names: 1-Docosanol

Bentonite (BEN-tow-nyt)

Definition: Bentonite is a native aluminum silicate clay that swells in the presence of water to produce a thick gel.
Class: Hydrous Aluminum Silicates
Function: Thickener, Emulsion Stabilizer, Suspending Agent, Absorbent
Found in: Hair Straighteners, Miscellaneous
Other Names: Soap Clay, CL 77004

Benzaldehyde (ben-ZAL-duh-hyd)

Definition: Benzaldehyde is an aromatic aldehyde.
Class: Aldehydes
Function: Fragrance
Found in: Miscellaneous

Other Names: Artificial Almond Oil, Benzenecarbonal, Benzoic
Aldehyde, Phenylformaldehyde, Phylmethanol Aldehyde

Benzalkonium Chloride (ben-ZAHL-koh-nee-um KLOHR-yde)

Definition: Benzalkonium chloride is a mixture of alkylben-
zyldimethylammonium chlorides including lauryl, myristyl,
and cetyl alkyls.

Class: Quaternary Ammonium Compounds

Function: Surfactants—Foam Booster, Conditioners—
Antistatic, Biocide

Found in: Shampoos, Conditoners, Miscellaneous

Other Names: Alkyl Dimethyl Benzyl Ammonium Chloride

Benzoic Acid (BEN-zoh-ic AS-ud)

Definition: Benzoic acid is an aromatic acid.

Class: Carboxylic Acids

Function: Fragrance, pH Adjuster, Preservative

Found in: Shampoos, Conditioners, Miscellaneous

Other Names: Benzenecarboxylic Acid, Benzeneformic Acid

Benzophenone (BEN-zoh-feh-nohwn)

Definition: Benzophenone is an organic compound used to
absorb ultraviolet light.

Class: Benzophenones

Function: Sunscreen, Fragrance

Found in: Miscellaneous

Other Names: Diphenyl Ketone, Diphenylmethanone, Phenyl
Ketone

Benzyl Alcohol (BEN-zyl AL-kuh-hawl)

Definition: Benzyl alcohol is an aromatic alcohol that slowly
oxidizes to benzaldehyde.

Class: Alcohols

Function: Preservative, Fragrance, External Analgesic

Found in: Miscellaneous

Other Names: Benzenemethanol, Phenylcarbinol,
Phenylmethanol

B

Betaine (BEE-tain)

Definition: Betaine is derived from trimethylglycine and was first discovered in sugar beet molasses. Betaine is an inner salt, or zwitterion, because it contains both positive and negative charges.

Class: Betaines

Function: Conditioners — Humectants

Found in: Shampoo, Conditioner, Miscellaneous

Other Names: Trimethylglycine

BHA

Definition: BHA is a mixture of isomers of tertiary butyl-substituted 4-methoxyphenols that inhibits the oxidation and deterioration of oils and fats, and prevents them from becoming rancid.

Class: Phenols

Function: Antioxidant, Fragrance

Found in: Miscellaneous

Other Names: Butylated Hydroxyanisole

BHT

Definition: BHT is a substituted toluene that inhibits the oxidation and deterioration of oils and fats, and prevents them from becoming rancid.

Class: Phenols

Function: Antioxidant

Found in: Miscellaneous

Other Names: Butylated Hydroxytoluene

Biotin (BY-oh-tin)

Definition: Biotin is a crystalline acid that forms part of the vitamin B complex.

Class: Carboxylic Acids

Function: Conditioner

Found in: Shampoos, Conditioners, Miscellaneous

Other Names: Coenzyme R, Vitamin B7, Vitamin H

B

Bismuth Oxychloride (BIS-muth ahk-sy-KLOHR-eyed)
Definition: Bismuth oxychloride is an inorganic pigment.
Class: Colorants, Inorganic Salts
Function: Hair Colorant
Found in: Hair Dyes, Hair Colorants
Other Names: Pearl Supreme, Pearl White, Pigment White 14, Chlorbismol

Blue 1 (BLOO)
Definition: Blue 1 is a triphenylmethane colorant.
Class: Colorants
Function: Colorant
Found in: Shampoos, Conditioner, Miscellaneous
Other Names: FD&C Blue No.1

Boric Acid (BOR-ik AS-ud)
Definition: Boric acid is an inorganic acid that has antibacterial and antifungal properties.
Class: Inorganic Acids
Function: Preservative, pH Adjuster
Found in: Shampoos, Conditioners, Miscellaneous
Other Names: Boron Trihydroxide, Trihydroxyborane

Brown 1 (BROUN)
Definition: Brown 1 is a diazo color.
Class: Colorants
Function: Hair Colorant
Found in: Hair Dyes, Hair Colorants
Other Names: D&C Brown No. 1

Butane (BYOOT-ayn)
Definition: Butane is a colorless, inflammable hydrocarbon gas.
Class: Hydrocarbons
Function: Propellant
Found in: Aerosol Hairspray
Other Names: n-Butane

B

Butoxydiglycol (BYOOT-ahk-si-dy-gly-kawl)

Definition: Butoxydiglycol is an ether alcohol used as a fragrance.

Class: Alcohols, Ethers

Function: Fragrance

Found in: Miscellaneous

Other Names: Butyl Carbitol, Butyl Diglycol, Butyl Dioxitol

Butyl Acetate (BYOOT-ul AS-uh-tayt)

Definition: Butyl acetate is the ester of butyl alcohol and acetic acid.

Class: Esters

Function: Fragrance

Found in: Miscellaneous

Other Names: Butyl Ethanoate

Butylene Glycol (BYOOT-ul-een GLY-kawl)

Definition: Butylene glycol is an aliphatic diol that is similar to propylene glycol. It is used as a solvent for many plant extracts.

Class: Alcohols

Function: Fragrance, Conditioners—Humectant, Thickener

Found in: Shampoos, Conditioners, Miscellaneous

Other Names: 1,3 Butanediol, 1,3 Dihydroxybutane

Butyl Ester of PVM/MA Copolymer (BYOOT-ul ES-ter KOH-pahl-uh-mur)

Definition: Butyl Ester of PVM/MA Copolymer is a polymer of the butyl ester of the polycarboxylic resin formed from vinyl methyl ether and maleic anhydride.

Class: Esters, Synthetic Polymers

Function: Hair Fixative, Film Former

Found in: Hairsprays, Aerosol Hairsprays

Other Names: Vinyl Methyl Ether Butyl Maleate Copolymer

Butylparaben (BYOOT-ul-par-uh-ben)

Definition: Butylparaben is the ester of butyl alcohol and p-hydroxybenzoic acid.

Class: Esters, Phenols

Function: Preservative

Found in: Shampoos, Conditioners, Miscellaneous

Other Names: Butyl Parahydroxybenzoate, Parahydroxybenzoate Ester

Butyl Stearate (BYOOT-ul STEER-ayt)

Definition: Butyl stearate is the ester of butyl alcohol and stearic acid.

Class: Esters

Function: Fragrance, Conditioner

Found in: Shampoos, Conditioners, Miscellaneous

Other Names: Octadecanoic Acid, Butyl Ester

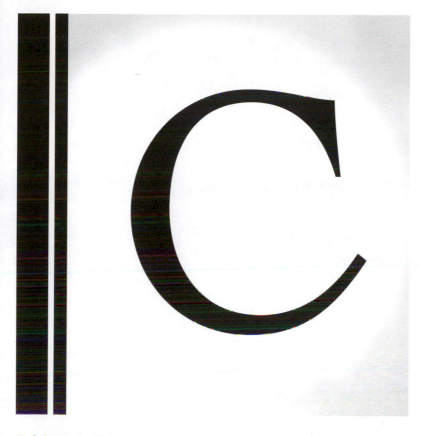

Calcium Carbonate (KAL-see-um KAR-bon-ayt)
  Definition: Calcium carbonate is an inorganic salt.
  Class: Inorganic Salt
  Function: pH Adjuster, Abrasive
  Found in: Depilatories
  Other Names: Heavy Calcium Carbonate, Precipitated Chalk

Calcium Chloride (KAL-see-um KHLOR-eyed)
  Definition: Calcium chloride is an inorganic salt.
  Class: Inorganic Salt
  Function: Thickener, Astingent
  Found in: Shampoos, Conditioners, Miscellaneous
  Other Names: Calcium Dichloride, Calcium Chloride, Dihydrate

C

Calcium Disodium EDTA (KAL-see-um DY-soh-dee-um)

Definition: Calcium disodium EDTA is a substituted diamine.
Class: Alkyl-Substituted Amino Acids, Amines, Organic Salts
Function: Chelating Agent
Found in: Shampoos, Conditioners, Miscellaneous
Other Names: Calcium Disodium Ethylenediamine Tetraacetate

Calcium Hydroxide (KAL-see-um hy-DRAHKS-eyed)

Definition: Calcium hydroxide is an inorganic alkali.
Class: Inorganic Alkali
Function: pH Adjuster
Found in: Hair Straightening—Hydroxide Relaxers, Depilatories, Miscellaneous
Other Names: Lime Water, Hydrated Lime, Calcium Hydrate, Calcium Dihydroxide

Calcium Oxide (KAL-see-um AHKS-eyed)

Definition: Calcium oxide is an inorganic oxide.
Class: Inorganics
Function: pH Adjuster
Found in: Miscellaneous
Other Names: Calcia, Calcium Monoxide, Lime

Calcium Pantothenate (KAL-see-um PAN-tow-thu-nayt)

Definition: Calcium pantothenate is a calcium salt of pantothenic acid.
Class: Organic Salts
Function: Conditioner
Found in: Shampoos, Conditioners, Miscellaneous
Other Names: Pantothenic Acid Calcium Salt, Vitamin B-5 Calcium Salt

Calcium Peroxide (KAL-see-um pur-AHK-seyed)

Definition: Calcium peroxide is an inorganic oxide used as an oxidizing agent.

Class: Inorganics
Function: Oxidizers
Found in: Hair Dyes, Hair Colorants, Bleaches
Other Names: Calcium Dioxide

Calcium Thioglycolate (KAL-see-um thy-oh-GLY-kuh-layt)

Definition: Calcium thioglycolate is the calcium salt of thio-
glycolic acid.
Class: Organic Salts, Thio Compounds
Function: Depilating Agent
Found in: Depilatories
Other Names: Calcium Mercaptoacetate

C14-15 Alcohols (AL-kuh-hawls)

Definition: C14-15 alcohols is a mixture of synthetic fatty al-
cohols with 14 to 15 carbons in the alkyl chain.
Class: Fatty Alcohols
Function: Conditioner, Emollient, Thickener
Found in: Shampoos, Conditioners, Miscellaneous
Other Names: Alcohols C14-15

Calendula Extract (KAL-en-doo-lah EKS-trakt)

Definition: Calendula extract is an extract of the flowers of
Calendula officinalis.
Class: Biological Products
Function: Conditioner
Found in: Shampoos, Conditioners, Miscellaneous
Other Names: Marigold Extract, *Calendula officinalis* Flower
Extract

C12-15 Alkyl Benzoate (AL-kul BEN-zo-ayt)

Definition: C12-15 alkyl benzoate is the ester of benzoic acid
and C12-15 alcohols.
Class: Esters
Function: Conditioners — Moisturizer
Found in: Miscellaneous
Other Names: Alkyl Benzoate

Canola Oil (KAN-oh-lah OYL)

Definition: Canola oil is low erucic acid *Brassica campestris* (Rapeseed) Oil.

Class: Oil

Function: Conditioners—Moisturizer

Found in: Shampoos, Conditioners, Miscellaneous

Other Names: Low Erucic Acid Rapeseed Oil

Capric Acid (KAP-rik AS-ud)

Definition: Capric acid is an aliphatic fatty acid. The soap functions as a surfactant and cleansing agent.

Class: Fatty Acids

Function: Fragrance, Surfactants—Cleansing Agent

Found in: Miscellaneous

Other Names: Caprinic Acid, Caprynic Acid, Decanoic Acid, Decylic Acid

Caprylic/Capric Glyceride (KAP-ril-ik/KAP-rik GLIS-ur-eyed)

Definition: Caprylic/capric glyceride is a mixture of mono-, di-, and triglycerides of caprylic and capric acids.

Class: Glyceryl Esters

Function: Conditioners—Moisturizer

Found in: Shampoos, Conditioners, Miscellaneous

Other Names: Glycerides C8-10

Caramel (KAHR-uh-mel)

Definition: Caramel is the concentrated solution obtained from heating solutions of sucrose or glucose.

Class: Colorants, Carbohydrates

Function: Colorant

Found in: Hair Dyes, Hair Colorants, Shampoos, Conditioners, Miscellaneous

Other Names: Natural Brown 10

Carbomer (KAHR-buh-mer)

Definition: Carbomer is a polymer of acrylic acid cross-linked with an allyl ether of pentaerythritol, sucrose, or propylene.

Class: Synthetic Polymer
Function: Thickener, Stabilizer
Found in: Miscellaneous
Other Names: Carbomer 910, Carboxyvinylpolymer

Carbon Black (KAHR-bun BLAK)

Definition: Carbon black is a color composed of particles of elemental carbon obtained by incomplete combustion of hydrocarbons.
Class: Colorants
Function: Colorant
Found in: Miscellaneous
Other Names: Channel Black, Pigment Black 6

Carica Papaya Fruit Extract (KAHR-ih-ka pa-PY-uh FROOT EKS-trakt)

Definition: Carica papaya fruit extract is an extract of the fruit of the papaya *Carica papaya*.
Class: Biological Products
Function: Conditioner
Found in: Shampoos, Conditioners, Miscellaneous
Other Names: Papaya Extract

Carmine (KAHR-myn)

Definition: Carmine is the aluminum lake of the coloring agent cochineal. Cochineal is the natural pigment derived from the dried female insect *Coccus cacti*.
Class: Colorants
Function: Colorant
Found in: Hair Dyes, Hair Colorants, Miscellaneous
Other Names: Carminic Acid, Carmine 5297, Natural Red 4

Carnitine (KAHR-nah-teen)

Definition: Carnitine is an organic compound that performs many different functions.
Class: Betaines

Function: Conditioners—Antistatic, Surfactant—Cleansing
   Agents, Thickener
Found in: Miscellaneous
Other Names: None Available

Carotene (KAIR-uh-tun)

Definition: Carotene is a carotenoid compound prepared syn-
   thetically or obtained from natural sources.
Class: Colorant
Function: Colorant
Found in: Miscellaneous
Other Names: Beta-Carotene, Food Orange 5, Natural Yel-
   low 26

Carthamus Tinctorius (Safflower) Seed Oil (KAHR-thu-mus TINK-tohr-ee-us SEED OYL)

Definition: Carthamus tinctorius (safflower) seed oil is the
   oily liquid obtained from the seeds of *Carthamus tinctorius.*
   It consists of the triglycerides of linoleic acid.
Class: Oils
Function: Conditioners—Moisturizer
Found in: Shampoos, Conditioners, Miscellaneous
Other Names: Safflower Oil, Safflower Seed Oil

Cellulose (SEL-yoo-lohs)

Definition: Cellulose is a natural polysaccharide derived from
   plant fibers.
Class: Biological Polymers
Function: Thickener, Absorbent
Found in: Shampoos, Conditioners, Miscellaneous
Other Names: Cellulose Powder, Wood Pulp, Bleached Wood
   Pulp

Ceramide 2 (SER-am-eyed)

Definition: Ceramide 2 is a synthetic N-acylated sphingold.
Class: Alcohols, Amides
Function: Conditioner

Found in: Shampoos, Conditioners, Miscellaneous
Other Names: 1-Steroyl-C-18 Sphingosine

C

Ceresin (SER-uh-sin)
Definition: Ceresin is a white to yellow waxy mixture of hydrocarbons obtained by purification of ozokerite.
Class: Waxes
Function: Thickener, Epilating Agent
Found in: Hair Dyes, Hair Colorants, Miscellaneous
Other Names: Cirine Wax, Mineral Wax, White Ozokerite Wax

Cetereth 3 (SET-ar-eth)
Definition: Cetereth 3 is the polyethylene glycol ether of cetyl alcohol condensed with 3 moles of ethylene oxide.
Class: Alkoxylated Alcohols
Function: Surfactants—Emulsifying Agent
Found in: Shampoos, Conditioners, Miscellaneous
Other Names: PEG-3 Cetyl/Stearyl Ether, Polyethylene Glycol (3) Cetyl/Stearyl Ether

Ceteryl Alcohol (SET-ear-ul AL-kuh-hawl)
Definition: Ceteryl alcohol is a mixture of cetyl alcohol (hexadecanol) and stearyl (octadecanol) alcohols.
Class: Fatty Alcohols
Function: Surfactants—Foam Booster, Thickeners
Found in: Miscellaneous
Other Names: Cetostearyl Alcohol, C16-18 Alcohol

Ceteth 2 (SET-eth)
Definition: Ceteth 2 is the polyethylene glycol ether of cetyl alcohol.
Class: Alkoxylated Alcohols
Function: Surfactants—Emulsifying Agent
Found in: Shampoos, Conditioners, Miscellaneous
Other Names: PEG-2

C

Cetoleth-6 (SET-oh-leth)

Definition: Cetoleth-6 is the polyethylene glycol ether of a mixture of cetyl alcohol and oleyl alcohol.

Class: Alkoxylated alcohols

Function: Surfactants — Emulsifying Agent

Found in: Shampoos, Conditioners, Miscellaneous

Other Names: PEG-6 Cetyl/Oleyl Ether

Cetrimonium Bromide (seh-tra-MOH-nee-um BRO-myd)

Definition: Cetrimonium bromide is a quaternary ammonium salt.

Class: Quaternary Ammonium Compounds

Function: Conditioners — Antistatic, Biocide, Surfactants — Emulsifying Agent

Found in: Hair Conditioners, Miscellaneous

Other Names: Cetyl Trimethyl Ammonium Bromide, CETAB

Cetrimonium Chloride (she-tra-MOH-nee-um KLOHR-eyed)

Definition: Cetrimonium chloride is a quaternary ammonium salt.

Class: Quaternary Ammonium Compounds

Function: Conditioners — Antistatic, Biocide, Surfactants — Emulsifying Agent

Found in: Shampoos, Conditioners, Permanent Waves, Hair Dyes, Hair Colorants, Miscellaneous

Other Names: Cetyl Trimethyl Ammonium Chloride

Cetyl Acetate (SEET-uhl AS-uh-tayt)

Definition: Cetyl acetate is the ester of cetyl alcohol and acetic acid.

Class: Esters

Function: Fragrance, Conditioner

Found in: Shampoos, Hairsprays, Miscellaneous

Other Names: 1-Acetoxyhexadecane, 1-Hexadecanol, Acetate

Cetyl Alcohol (SEET-uhl AL-kuh-hawl)

Definition: Cetyl alcohol was first discovered in 1813, and is the oldest and one of the most commonly used fatty alcohols. Originally found in large amounts in spermaceti wax from the sperm whale, natural cetyl alcohol is now obtained by hydrogenation of tallow. Commercial grades also contain myristyl alcohol and stearyl alcohol.

Class: Fatty Alcohols

Function: Surfactants—Emulsifying Agents, Surfactants—Foam Booster, Thickener

Found in: Shampoos, Conditioners, Miscellaneous

Other Names: Cetanol, 1-Hexadecanol, Palmityl Alcohol, C-16 Alcohol

Cetyl Palmitate (SEET-uhl PAL-muh-tayt)

Definition: Cetyl palmitate is the ester of cetyl alcohol and palmitic acid.

Class: Esters

Function: Fragrance, Conditioners—Moisturizer

Found in: Shampoos, Conditioners, Miscellaneous

Other Names: Hexadecyl Palmitate, Hexadecanoic Acid, Hexadecyl Ester

Chamomilla Recutita (Matricaria) Flower Extract (KAM-oh-me-lah REK-ooh-tea-sha FLOW-ur EKS-trakt)

Definition: Chamomilla recutita (matricaria) extract is an extract of *Chamomile recutita* (German chamomile). Chamomile has been used medicinally for centuries. Its anti-inflammatory properties are due to the chemical chamazule. Chamomile also contains azulene, which is an intensely blue compound used to brighten hair.

Class: Biological Products

Function: Conditioner

Found in: Shampoos, Conditioners, Hair Dyes, Hair Colorants, Miscellaneous

Other Names: Camomille Extract, Chamomile Extract, German Chamomile Extract

Chitosan (KEYE-tow-san)

Definition: Chitosan is a deacylated derivative of chitin. Chitin is a glucosamine polysaccharide derived from the shells of crabs, lobsters, and beetles.
Class: Biological Polymers
Function: Chelating Agent, Film Former
Found in: Hair Grooming Aids
Other Names: Deacetylchitin

Cholecalciferol (KOHL-uh-kal-sif-ur-awl)

Definition: Cholecalciferol is a vitamin that occurs in fish liver oils and is synthesized in the human body by sunlight on the skin. It is unlikely that small amounts added to cosmetics are beneficial.
Class: Alcohols, Sterols
Function: Conditioner
Found in: Shampoos, Conditioners, Permanent Waves, Miscellaneous
Other Names: Arachitol, Vitamin D-3

Cholesterol (koh-LES-tur-awl)

Definition: Cholesterol is the mono-unsaturated sterol that is found in human sebum and all animal body tissues. Lanolin is high in cholesterol. The lanolin alcohol obtained from wool grease contains 25 percent to 30 percent cholesterol.
Class: Alcohols, Sterols
Function: Conditioners—Moisturizer, Emulsion Stabilizer, Thickener
Found in: Shampoos, Conditioners, Hairsprays, Setting Lotions, Hair Dyes, Hair Colorants, Miscellaneous
Other Names: Cholesterin, Cholesteryl Alcohol, Provitamin D

Choleth-5 (koh-LETH)

Definition: Choleth-5 is a polyethylene glycol ether of cholesterol with an average ethoxylation value of 5.

Class: Alkoxylated Alcohols, Sterols

Function: Surfactants—Emulsifying Agent

Found in: Shampoos, Conditioners, Hair Dyes, Hair Colorants, Miscellaneous

Other Names: Polyethylene Glycol (5) Cholesteryl Ether

Citric Acid (SIT-rik AS-ud)

Definition: Citric acid is an organic acid that is found in fruits, especially citrus fruits (lemons, limes, and oranges).

Class: Carboxylic Acids

Function: Chelating Agent, Fragrance, pH Adjuster

Found in: Shampoos, Conditioners, Hairsprays, Setting Lotions, Hair Dyes, Hair Colorants, Miscellaneous

Other Names: Anhydrous Citric Acid, Citric Acid Monohydrate

Coal Tar (KOHL TAR)

Definition: Coat tar is a thick liquid or semi-solid obtained as a byproduct in the destructive distillation of bituminous coal. It contains many aromatic hydrocarbons, phenolic substances, and other compounds including benzene, xylene, toluene, cresol, naphthalene, and anthracene. In the United States, coal tar may be used as an active ingredient in over-the-counter drug products.

Class: Hydrocarbons

Function: Antidandruff Agent

Found in: Antidandruff Shampoos, Medicated Shampoos

Other Names: Tar, Coal

Cocamide DEA (koh-KUH-myd)

Definition: Cocamide DEA is a mixture of ethanol amides of coconut acid.

Class: Alkanolamides

Function: Surfactants—Foam Booster, Thickener

Found in: Shampoos, Conditioners, Hairsprays, Setting Lotions, Hair Dyes, Hair Colorants, Miscellaneous

Other Names: Cocamide Diethanolamide, Coconut Diethanolamide, Cocoyl Diethanolamide

Cocamide MEA (koh-KUH-myd)

Definition: Cocamide MEA is a mixture of ethanol amides of coconut acid. Cocamide MEA is similar to cocamide DEA, but is used only where its superior thickening properties are desired.

Class: Alkanolamides

Function: Surfactants—Foam Booster, Thickener

Found in: Shampoos, Conditioners, Hairsprays, Setting Lotions, Hair Dyes, Hair Colorants, Miscellaneous

Other Names: Cocamide Monoethanolamide, Coco Monoethanolamide, Cocoyl Monoethanolamide

Cocamidopropyl Betaine (koh-KUH-my-doh-pro-pil BEE-tayn)

Definition: Cocamidopropyl betaine is a zwitterion (inner salt) or pseudoamphoteric surfactant that is widely used to perform many different functions. It is a good conditioner because at an acidic pH, its cationic character makes it substantive to hair. It also aids in the deposition of proteins and cationic polymers on the hair. "Ringing Gels" can be formed when used with surfactants such as TEA-lauryl sulfate. Because cocamidopropyl betaine also reduces the irritation of other surfactants, it is frequently used in combination with a sulfate and a polysorbate in baby shampoos.

Class: Betaines

Function: Conditioners—Antistatic, Surfactants—Cleansing Agent, Foam Booster, Thickener

Found in: Shampoos, Conditioners, Hairsprays, Setting Lotions, Hair Dyes, Hair Colorants, Miscellaneous

Other Names: Cocamidopropyl Dimethyl Glycine, Cocoyl
Amide Propylbetaine

Cocamidopropyl Dimethylamine (koh-KUH-my-doh-pro-pil dy-meth-ul-AM-een)

Definition: Cocamidopropyl Dimethylamine is an ami-
doamine derived from coconut oil.

Class: Amines

Function: Conditioners — Antistatic

Found in: Shampoos, Conditioners, Miscellaneous

Other Names: Dimethylamino Propyl Coco Amides

Cocamidopropyl Hydroxysultaine (koh-KUH-my-doh-pro-pil hy-DRAHKS-ee-suhl-tayn)

Definition: Cocamidopropyl hydroxysultaine is a zwitterion
or pseudoamphoteric surfactant.

Class: Betaines

Function: Conditioners — Antistatic, Surfactants — Cleansing
Agent, Foam Booster, Thickener

Found in: Shampoos, Baby Shampoos, Conditioners,
Miscellaneous

Other Names: Cocamidopropyl Hydroxy Sulfopropyl Dimethyl Quaternary Ammonium Compounds

Coco-Betaine (koh-koh-BEE-tayn)

Definition: Coco-Betaine is a zwitterion or pseudoamphoteric
surfactant derived from coconut oil. It is mild and reduces
the irritation of other surfactants. It has good foaming
properties, is substantive to the hair, and provides antistatic and conditioning properties.

Class: Betaines

Function: Conditioners — Antistatic, Surfactants — Cleansing
Agent, Foam Booster, Thickener

Found in: Shampoos, Baby Shampoos, Conditioners,
Miscellaneous

Other Names: Coco Dimethyl Glycine, Coconut Betaine

Coconut Acid (KOH-kuh-nut AS-ud)

Definition: Coconut acid is a mixture of lauric, myristic, and palmitic fatty acids derived from coconut oil.

Class: Fatty Acids

Function: Surfactants—Cleansing Agent

Found in: Shampoos, Miscellaneous

Other Names: Coco Fatty Acid, Coconut Oil Acids

Cocoyl Sarcosine (KOH-koil sar-KOH-seen)

Definition: Cocoyl sarcosine is the N-cocoyl derivative of sarcosine derived from coconut oil.

Class: Sarcosinates

Function: Surfactants—Cleansing Agent, Conditioner

Found in: Shampoos, Conditioners, Miscellaneous

Other Names: Cocoyl Sarcosine, Cocoyl Methyl Glycine

Collagen (KAHL-uh-jen)

Definition: Collagen is a large, cross-linked protein found in the cartilage and other connective tissues of animals. Low molecular weight collagen derivatives are usually used in cosmetics because their smaller size makes them more soluble and substantive to the hair.

Class: Proteins

Function: Conditioners

Found in: Shampoos, Conditioners, Hairsprays, Setting Lotions, Hair Dyes, Hair Colorants, Miscellaneous

Other Names: Collagen Fiber, Collagen Sheet

C11-15 Pareth-7 (PAR-eth)

Definition: C11-15 Pareth-7 is a polyethylene glycol ether of a mixture of synthetic C11-15 fatty alcohols with an average ethoxylation value of 5.

Class: Alkoxylated Alcohols

Function: Surfactants—Emulsifying Agent

Found in: Shampoos, Conditioners, Miscellaneous

Other Names: Pareth-15-7

Curry Red (Kur-ee RED)
Definition: Curry red is an organic monoazo color.
Class: Colorants
Function: Colorant
Found in: Shampoos, Conditioners, Hairsprays, Miscellaneous
Other Names: Allura Red AC, CL 16035, Food Red 17

Cyclodextrin (sy-kloh-DEKS-trin)
Definition: Cyclodextrin is a cyclic polysaccharide comprised of six to eight glucopyranose units.
Class: Carbohydrates
Function: Chelating Agents
Found in: Shampoos, Conditioners, Miscellaneous
Other Names: Alphadex, Betadex, Cycloamylose

Cycloheptasiloxane (sy-kloh-hep-tuh-sy-LOHKS-ayn)
Definition: Cycloheptasiloxane is a cyclic dimethyl polysiloxane.
Class: Siloxanes, Silanes
Function: Conditioners—Emollient
Found in: Hair Conditioners, Hairsprays, Hair Dyes, Hair Colorants
Other Names: Cycloheptasiloxane Tetradecamethylcyclomethicone

Cyclomethicone (sy-kloh-METH-ah-kohn)
Definition: Cyclomethicone is a generic name for cyclic dimethyl polysiloxane compounds commonly called silicones.
Class: Siloxanes and Silanes
Function: Conditioners—Moisturizer
Found in: Shampoos, Conditioners, Hairsprays, Setting Lotions, Hair Dyes, Hair Colorants, Miscellaneous
Other Names: Methylcyclopolysiloxane

Cysteamine HCL (SIS-tee-uh-meen)
Definition: Cysteamine HCL is an amine salt.
Class: Organic Salts, Thio Compounds

C

Function: Hair Waving and Straightening—Reducing Agent

Found in: Permanent Waves, Hair Straighteners

Other Names: Aminoethanethiol Hydrochloride, Cysteamine Hydrochloride

Cysteine (SIS-tuh-een)

Definition: Cysteine is a naturally occurring amino acid found in hair and skin.

Class: Amino Acids, Thio Compounds

Function: Hair Waving and Straightening—Reducing Agent, Conditioner

Found in: Permanent Waves, Hair Straighteners, Conditioners, Miscellaneous

Other Names: L-Cysteine, Cysteine DL

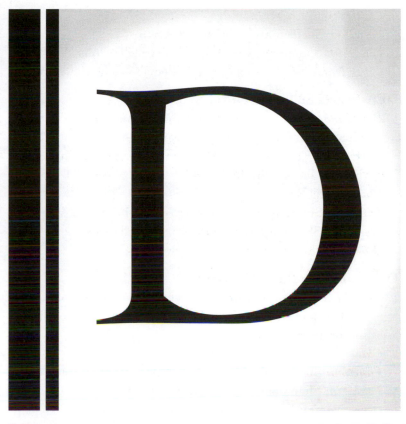

DEA: *See* **Diethanolamine**

DEA-C12-13 Alkyl Sulfate (AL-kil SUL-fayt)

Definition: DEA-C12-13 alkyl sulfate is the diethanolamine salt of the sulfate of C12-13 alcohols.

Class: Alkyl Sulfates

Function: Surfactants—Cleansing Agent

Found in: Shampoos, Conditioners, Miscellaneous

Other Names: Diethanolamine Alkyl Sulfate

DEA-Dodecylbenzenesulfonate (doh-dek-il-ben-zeen-SUL-fuh-nayt)

Definition: DEA-Dodecylbenzenesulfonate is the diethanolamine salt of Dodecylbenzene sulfonic acid.

Class: Alkyl Aryl Sulfonates
Function: Surfactants—Cleansing Agent
Found in: Shampoos, Conditioners, Miscellaneous
Other Names: Diethanolamine Dodecylbenzene Sulfonate

DEA-Lauryl Sulfate (LOR-ul SUL-fayt)

Definition: DEA-lauryl sulfate is the diethanolamine salt of lauryl sulfate where "lauryl" means predominantly C12-14 alcohols. This is an excellent cleansing and foaming agent that produces rich, thick suds.
Class: Alkyl Sulfates
Function: Surfactants—Cleansing Agent, Foam Booster
Found in: Shampoos, Conditioners, Miscellaneous
Other Names: Diethanolamine Lauryl Sulfate

DEA-Linoleate (lin-OH-lee-ayt)

Definition: DEA-linoleate is the diethanolamine salt of linoleic acid. It is a very soluble soap with good conditioning properties.
Class: Soaps
Function: Surfactants—Cleansing Agent, Conditioner
Found in: Shampoos, Conditioners, Miscellaneous
Other Names: Diethanolamine Linoleate

DEA-Methoxycinnamate (meth-ahk-see-SIN-uh-mayt)

Definition: DEA-methoxycinnamate is the diethanolamine salt of methoxycinnamic acid.
Class: Ethers, Organic Salts
Function: Sunscreen
Found in: Shampoos, Conditioners, Hairsprays, Setting Lotions
Other Names: Diethanolamine Methoxycinnamate

DEA-Oleth-10 Phosphate (OH-leth FAHS-fayt)

Definition: DEA-oleth-10 phosphate is the diethanolamine salt of a complex mixture of oleth-10 phosphate.
Class: Phosphorus Compounds

D

Function: Surfactants — Emulsifying Agent
Found in: Shampoos, Conditioners, Permanent Waves, Hair Straighteners, Miscellaneous
Other Names: Diethanolamine Oleth-10 Phosphate

Decanal (dek-UH-nal)

Definition: Decanal is an aldehyde use as a fragrance additive.
Class: Aldehydes
Function: Fragrance
Found in: Shampoos, Conditioners, Miscellaneous
Other Names: Capric Aldehyde, Decyl Aldehyde

Deceth-8 (DEK-eth)

Definition: Deceth-8 is the polyethylene glycol ether of decyl alcohol with an average value of 8.
Class: Alkoxylated Alcohols
Function: Surfactants — Emulsifying Agent
Found in: Shampoos, Conditioners, Miscellaneous
Other Names: PEG-8 Decyl Ether, Polyethylene Glycol 400 Decyl Ether, Polyoxyethylene (8) Decyl Ether

Deceth-4 Phosphate (DEK-eth FAHS-fayt)

Definition: Deceth-4 phosphate is a complex mixture of phosphoric acid ester of Deceth-4.
Class: Phosphorus Compounds
Function: Surfactants — Emulsifying Agent
Found in: Shampoos, Conditioners, Miscellaneous
Other Names: PEG-4 Decyl Ether Phosphate, Polyethylene Glycol 200 Decyl Ether Phosphate

Decyl Alcohol (DEK-il AL-kuh-hawl)

Definition: Decyl alcohol is a fatty alcohol.
Class: Fatty Alcohol
Function: Fragrance, Surfactants — Foam Booster, Thickener
Found in: Shampoos, Conditioners, Miscellaneous
Other Names: 1-Decanol, n-Decanol, 1-Hydroxydecane

D

Decyl Oleate (DEK-il OH-lee-ayt)
>   *Definition:* Decyl oleate is the ester of decyl alcohol and oleic acid.
>   *Class:* Esters
>   *Function:* Conditioners—Moisturizer
>   *Found in:* Shampoos, Conditioners, Hair Dyes, Hair Colorants, Miscellaneous
>   *Other Names:* Decyl-9-Octadecanoate

Dehydroacetic Acid (dee-hy-droh-AS-eh-tik AS-ud)
>   *Definition:* Dehydroacetic acid is a cyclic ketone used as a bactericide and fungicide.
>   *Class:* Carboxylic Acids, Heterocyclic Compounds
>   *Function:* Preservative
>   *Found in:* Shampoos, Conditioners, Miscellaneous
>   *Other Names:* 3-acetyl-6-methyl-1,2-pyran-2,4 dione

Dextrin (DEKS-trin)
>   *Definition:* Dextrin is a gum produced by the incomplete hydrolysis of starch.
>   *Class:* Gums, Colloids
>   *Function:* Thickener, Absorbent
>   *Found in:* Hair Bleaches, Hair Lighteners with Color
>   *Other Names:* Dextrine

3,4-Diaminobenzoic Acid (dy-uh-MEE-noh BEN-zoh-ik AS-ud)
>   *Definition:* 3,4-diaminobenzoic acid is a substituted aromatic compound.
>   *Class:* Amino Acids
>   *Function:* Hair Colorant
>   *Found in:* Hair Dyes, Hair Colorants
>   *Other Names:* Benzoic Acid, 3,4 Diamino

4,4-Diaminodiphenylamine (dy-uh-MEE-noh-dy-feh-nil-ah-meen)
>   *Definition:* 4,4-diaminodiphenylamine is an aromatic amine hair colorant.

Class: Amines
Function: Hair Colorant
Found in: Hair Dyes, Hair Colorants
Other Names: 4,4-Iminodianiline

2,4-Diaminophenol (dy-uh-MEE-noh-feh-nawl)

Definition: 2,4-diaminophenol is an aromatic amine hair colorant.
Class: Amines, Phenols
Function: Hair Colorant
Found in: Hair Dyes, Hair Colorants
Other Names: Phenol, 2,4-Diamino

2,4-Diaminophenoxyethanol HCL (dy-uh-MEE-noh-fehn-ahk-see-eth-un-awl)

Definition: 2,4-diaminophenoxyethanol HCL is an aromatic amine salt.
Class: Amines
Function: Hair Colorant
Found in: Hair Dyes, Hair Colorants, Aerosol Hair Color Sprays
Other Names: Ethanol, 2 Dihydrochloride

2,6-Diaminopyridine (dy-uh-MEE-noh-pir-uh-deen)

Definition: 2,6-diaminopyridine is an aromatic amine hair colorant.
Class: Amines, Heterocyclic Compounds
Function: Hair Colorant
Found in: Hair Dyes, Hair Colorants
Other Names: 2,6-Pyridinediamine

Diammonium Lauryl Sulfosuccinate (dy-uh-MOH-nee-um LOR-ul SULF-oh-suk-ah-nayt)

Definition: Diammonium lauryl sulfosuccinate is the ammonium salt of a lauryl alcohol half ester of sulfosuccinic acid.
Class: Sulfosuccinates
Function: Surfactants—Cleansing Agent

Found in: Shampoos, Conditioners, Miscellaneous

Other Names: Sulfobutanedioic Acid, 1-Dodecyl Ester, Diammonium Salt

Diatomaceous Earth (dy-uh-TOM-ay-sush URTH)

D

Definition: Diatomaceous earth is a mineral consisting primarily of the silicone fragments of various species of diatoms.

Class: Inorganics

Function: Abrasive, Absorbent

Found in: Cleansing Products

Other Names: Diatomite, Siliceous Earth

Diazolidinyl Urea (dy-uh-ZOHL-id-in-il YUR-ee-uh)

Definition: Diazolidinyl urea is a heterocyclic substituted urea.

Class: Amides, Heterocyclic Compounds

Function: Preservative

Found in: Shampoos, Conditioners, Hairsprays, Setting Lotions, Hair Dyes, Hair Colorants, Miscellaneous

Other Names: Urea, N-2,5-Dioxo-4-Imidazolidinyl-N-N-Bis
Urea

Dicetyldimonium Chloride (dy-set-il-dy-MOH-nee-um KHLOR-eyed)

Definition: Dicetyldimonium chloride is a quaternary ammonium salt.

Class: Quaternary Ammonium Compounds

Function: Conditioners—Antistatic

Found in: Shampoos, Conditioners, Hairsprays, Setting Lotions, Hair Dyes, Hair Colorants, Miscellaneous

Other Names: Quaternium-31

Diethanolamine (dy-eth-an-all-AM-een)

Definition: Diethanolamine is an aliphatic amine.

Class: Alkanolamines

Function: pH Adjuster

Found in: Shampoos, Conditioners, Hair Dyes, Hair Colorants, Miscellaneous

Other Names: DEA, 2,2-Dihydroxydiethylamine

Diethylhexyl Sebacate (dy-eth-il-HEKS-il SEB-uh-sayt)

Definition: Diethylhexyl sebacate is the diester of 2-ethyl-hexyl alcohol and sebacic acid.

Class: Esters

Function: Fragrance, Solvent, Film Former

Found in: Hairsprays, Aerosol Hairsprays, Setting Lotions, Miscellaneous

Other Names: Dioctyl Sebacate

Diethylhexyl Sodium Sulfosuccinate (dy-eth-il-HEKS-il SOW-dee-um SULF-oh-suk-ah-nayt)

Definition: Diethylhexyl Sodium Sulfosuccinate is the sodium salt of the diester of 2-ethylhexyl alcohol and sulfosuccinic acid.

Class: Sulfosuccinates

Function: Surfactants—Cleansing Agent

Found in: Hair Bleaches, Miscellaneous

Other Names: Dioctyl Sodium Sulfosuccinate, Docusate Sodium

Diethyl Phthalate (dy -ETH-il THAL-ayt)

Definition: Diethyl phthalate is an aromatic diester of ethyl alcohol and phthalic acid.

Class: Esters

Function: Fragrance, Solvent

Found in: Hair Conditioners

Other Names: Diethyl 1,2-Benzenedicarboxylate

Dihydrogenated Tallow Benzylmonium Chloride (dy-hy-DROH-jen-ayt-ed TAL-oh ben-ZAHL-moh-nee-um KHLOR-eyed)

Definition: Dihydrogenated tallow benzylmonium chloride is a quaternary ammonium salt.

Class: Quaternary Ammonium Compounds

Function: Conditioners—Antistatic

Found in: Shampoos, Conditioners, Miscellaneous

Other Names: None Available

D

Dihydroxyethyl Cocamine Oxide (dy-hy-DRAHKS-ee-eth-ul KOH-kuh-myn AHKS-eyed)

Definition: Dihydroxyethyl cocamine oxide is a tertiary amine oxide derived from coconut oil.

Class: Amine Oxides

Function: Surfactants—Cleansing Agent, Foam Booster, Conditioner

Found in: Shampoos, Conditioners, Miscellaneous

Other Names: Amines, Coco Alkyl Dihydroxyethyl, Oxides

Dihydroxyethyl Tallow Glycinate (dy-hy-DRAHKS-ee-eth-ul TAL-oh GLY-sin-ayt)

Definition: Although it is not named as such, dihydroxyethyl tallow glycinate is actually a betaine derived from tallow.

Class: Alkyl-Substituted Amino Acids

Function: Conditioners—Moisturizer

Found in: Shampoos, Conditioners, Hair Dyes, Hair Colorants, Miscellaneous

Other Names: Tallow Dihydroxyethyl Betaine

Diisobutyl Adipate (dy-eye-soh-BYOOT-ul AD-ah-payt)

Definition: Diisobutyl adipate is the diester of isobutyl alcohol and adipic acid.

Class: Esters

Function: Solvent, Fragrance, Film Former

Found in: Hairsprays, Aerosol Hairsprays

Other Names: Diisobutyl Hexanedioate

Dimethicone (dy-METH-ah-kohn)

Definition: Dimethicone is a mixture of fully methylated linear siloxane polymers that are end-blocked with trimethylsiloxy units. Dimethicone refers to various blends of a series of polydimethylsiloxanes of varying viscosity. Dimethicones are nontacky lubricants used to impart a soft feel and a shiny, water-repellant, breathable film to hair.

Class: Siloxanes and Silanes

Function: Conditioner

Found in: Shampoos, Conditioners, Hairsprays, Setting Lotions, Hair Dyes, Hair Colorants, Permanent Waves and Hair Straighteners, Miscellaneous

Other Names: Dimethylpolysiloxane, Dimethyl Silicone, Silicone L-45

D

Dimethicone Copolyol (dy-METH-ah-kohn KOH-pah-lee-awl)

Definition: Dimethicone copolyol is a family of nonionic surfactants with varying degrees of solubility depending on their ethylene oxide content. Dimethicone copolyol is used to aid wet combing, provide softness, and reduce flyaway hair. Dimethicone copolyol does not build up on the hair because it is water-soluble.

Class: Siloxanes

Function: Surfactants—Emulsifying Agent, Conditioner

Found in: Shampoos, Conditioners, Hairsprays, Setting Lotions, Hair Dyes, Hair Colorants, Miscellaneous

Other Names: Dimethylsiloxane-Glycol Copolymer

Dimethiconol (dy-METH-ah-kon-awl)

Definition: Dimethiconol is a dimethyl siloxane terminated with hydroxyl groups.

Class: Siloxanes and Silanes

Function: Conditioner, Antifoaming Agent

Found in: Shampoos, Conditioners, Miscellaneous

Other Names: Dihydroxypolydimethylsiloxane

Dimethyl Behenamine (dy-METH-ul beh-hen-AM-een)

Definition: Dimethyl behenamine is a long chain, fatty, aliphatic, tertiary amine. This cationic emulsifying agent is used to soften and condition hair.

Class: Amines

Function: Conditioners—Antistatic

Found in: Shampoos, Conditioners, Miscellaneous

Other Names: Behenyl Dimethyl Amine, Dimethyl Beheny-
lamine, Docosyl Dimethylamine

Dimethyl Ether (dy-METH-ul EETH-ur)
Definition: Dimethyl ether is an organic compound.
Class: Ethers
Function: Propellant, Solvent
Found in: Hairsprays, Aerosol Hairsprays, Miscellaneous
Other Names: Dimethyl Oxide, Methoxymethane

Dimethyl Lauramine (dy-METH-ul LOR-am-een)
Definition: Dimethyl lauramine is a tertiary aliphatic amine.
Class: Amines
Function: Conditioners—Antistatic
Found in: Shampoos, Conditioners, Miscellaneous
Other Names: Dimethyl Laurylamine, Lauryl Dimethyl Amine

Dimethyl Lauramine Oleate (dy-METH-ul LOR-am-een OH-lee-ayt)
Definition: Dimethyl lauramine oleate is the salt of dimethyl
lauramine and oleic acid. This cationic conditioner imparts
long lasting slip and lubrication to hair.
Class: Amines
Function: Surfactants—Emulsifying Agent, Conditioner
Found in: Conditioners, Miscellaneous
Other Names: Lauryl Dimethylamine Oleate, Dodecyl Di-
methylamine Oleate

Dimethyl Octynediol (dy-METH-ul AHK-teen-dy-awl)
Definition: Dimethyl octynediol is an aliphatic alcohol. It is a
nonionic surfactant that is used to clarify and reduce or
control the thickness of the finished product.
Class: Alcohols
Function: Surfactants—Emulsifying Agent
Found in: Shampoos, Conditioners, Setting Lotions,
Miscellaneous
Other Names: 3,6-dimethyl-4-octyne-3,6-diol

D

Dimethyl Palmitamine (dy-METH-ul PAHL-mah-tam-een)

Definition: Dimethyl palmitamine is a tertiary aliphatic amine.
Class: Amines
Function: Conditioners—Antistatic
Found in: Shampoos, Conditioners, Miscellaneous
Other Names: Palmityl Dimethyl Amine

Dimethyl-p-Phenylenediamine (dy-METH-ul FEN-ahl-een-dy-am-een)

Definition: Dimethyl-p-phenylenediamine is a substituted aromatic amine hair colorant.
Class: Amines
Function: Hair Colorant
Found in: Hair Dyes, Hair Colorants
Other Names: 4-Dimethylamino Aniline, CL 76075

Dimethyl Stearamine (dy-METH-ul STEER-am-een)

Definition: Dimethyl stearamine is a tertiary aliphatic amine that is prepared from stearic acid. The neutral salt, which is cationic, softens and conditions hair, and has emulsifying properties.
Class: Amines
Function: Conditioners—Antistatic
Found in: Hairsprays, Aerosol Hairsprays, Hair Conditioners, Miscellaneous
Other Names: Stearyl Dimethyl Amine, Dymanthine, Dimethyl Octadecylamine

Dipentene (dy-PEN-teen)

Definition: Dipentene is a terpene that occurs naturally in many essential oils. Although it is a known irritant and allergen, it is believed to be harmless when used at low levels.
Class: Hydrocarbons
Function: Fragrance, Solvent
Found in: Shampoos, Conditioners, Miscellaneous
Other Names: Limonene

Dipropylene Glycol (dy-PRO-pahl-een GLY-kawl)

Definition: Dipropylene glycol is a mixture of diols used as a solvent to dissolve water insoluble ingredients. It is similar to propylene glycol and butylene glycol. It is irritating to the skin and is known to be more irritating than propylene glycol.

Class: Alcohols, Ethers

Function: Solvent, Fragrance

Found in: Shampoos, Conditioners, Hairsprays, Setting Lotions, Hair Dyes, Hair Colorants, Permanent Waves, Hair Straighteners, Miscellaneous

Other Names: 1,1-Dimethyldiethylene Glycol, 1,1-Oxybis-2-Propanol

Direct Black 51 (DY-rekt BLAK)

Definition: Direct black 51 is a diazo hair colorant.

Class: Hair Color Additives

Function: Hair Colorant

Found in: Hair Dyes, Hair Colorants

Other Names: Saturn Black B

Direct Blue 86 (DY-rekt BLOO)

Definition: Direct blue 86 is a phthalocyanine colorant.

Class: Hair Color Additives

Function: Colorant

Found in: Shampoos, Conditioners, Miscellaneous

Other Names: Heliogen Blue CL

Direct Red 80 (DY-rekt RED)

Definition: Direct red 80 is a polyazo hair colorant.

Class: Hair Color Additives

Function: Hair Colorant

Found in: Hair Dyes, Hair Colorants

Other Names: Saturn Red F 3B, Sirius Red F 3B

Direct Violet 48 (DY-rekt VY-let)

Definition: Direct violet 48 is a diazo hair colorant.

Class: Hair Color Additives
Function: Hair Colorant
Found in: Hair Dyes, Hair Colorants
Other Names: None Available

Direct Yellow 12 (DY-rekt YEL-oh)
Definition: Direct yellow 12 is a diazo color.
Class: Hair Color Additives
Function: Hair Colorant
Found in: Hair Dyes, Hair Colorants
Other Names: Chrysophenine

Disiloxane (dy-sy-LOHKS-ayn)
Definition: Disiloxane is a linear siloxane.
Class: Siloxanes and Silanes
Function: Conditioner
Found in: Hairsprays, Aerosol Hairsprays
Other Names: Bis Trimethyl Ether

Disodium Capryloamphodiacetate (dy-SOH-dee-um KAP-ril-oh-amp-foh-dy-as-uh-tayt)
Definition: Disodium capryloamphodiacetate is an ampho-teric surfactant.
Class: Alkylamido Alkylamines
Function: Surfactants—Cleansing Agent, Foam Booster, Conditioner
Found in: Shampoos, Conditioners, Miscellaneous
Other Names: Capryloamphocarboxyglycinate, Capryloamphodiacetate

Disodium Cocamido MEA-Sulfosuccinate (dy-SOH-dee-um KOH-kuh-my-doh sul-foh-SUHK-in-ayt)
Definition: Disodium cocamido MEA-sulfosuccinate is a dis-odium salt of a substituted ethanolamide half ester of sul-fosuccinic acid derived from coconut oil.
Class: Sulfosuccinates, Sulfosuccinamates
Function: Surfactants—Cleansing Agent

Found in: Shampoos, Conditioners, Miscellaneous
Other Names: Disodium Cocoylmonoethanolamide
Sulfosuccinate

Disodium Cocoamphodiacetate (dy-SOH-dee-um KOH-koh-amp-foh-dy-as-uh-tayt)

Definition: Disodium cocoamphodiacetate is an amphoteric
surfactant derived from coconut oil.
Class: Alkylamido Alkylamines
Function: Surfactants—Cleansing Agent, Foam Booster,
Conditioner
Found in: Shampoos, Hair Dyes, Hair Colorants,
Miscellaneous
Other Names: Cocoamphocarboxyglycinate,
Cocoamphodiacetate

Disodium Cocoamphodipropionate (dy-SOH-dee-um KOH-koh-amp-foh-dy-proh-pee-eye-ohn-tayt)

Definition: Disodium cocoamphodipropionate is an ampho-
teric surfactant derived from coconut oil.
Class: Alkylamido Alkylamines
Function: Surfactants—Cleansing Agent, Foam Booster,
Conditioner
Found in: Shampoos, Conditioners, Hair Dyes, Hair Col-
orants, Miscellaneous
Other Names: Cocoamphocarboxypropionate,
Cocoamphodipropionate

Disodium C12-15 Pareth Sulfosuccinate (dy-SOH-dee-um PAR-eth SUL-foh-sook-in-ayt)

Definition: Disodium C12-15 pareth sulfosuccinate is the
disodium salt of an ethoxylated, partially esterfied,
sulfosuccinic acid
Class: Sulfosuccinates, Sulfosuccinamates
Function: Surfactants—Cleansing Agent, Foam Booster
Found in: Shampoos, Conditioners, Miscellaneous
Other Names: Disodium Pareth-25 Sulfosuccinate

Disodium EDTA (dy-SOH-dee-um)

Definition: Disodium EDTA is a substituted diamine used as a chelating agent.

Class: Alkyl-Substituted Amino Acids

Function: Chelating Agent

Found in: Shampoos, Conditioners, Hairsprays, Setting Lotions, Permanent Waves, Hair Straighteners, Hair Dyes, Hair Colorants, Miscellaneous

Other Names: Disodium Edetate, Edetate Disodium, Disodium Ethylenediaminetetraacetate

Disodium EDTA-Copper (dy-SOH-dee-um KOP-ur)

Definition: Disodium EDTA-copper is a copper chelate of disodium EDTA.

Class: Alkyl-Substituted Amino Acids

Function: Colorant

Found in: Shampoos, Conditioners, Miscellaneous

Other Names: Copper Versenate, Disodium Cupric Ethylenediaminetetraacetate

Disodium Lauramido MEA-Sulfosuccinate (dy-SOH-dee-um LOHR-uh-my-doh SUL-foh-sook-in-ayt)

Definition: Disodium lauramido MEA-sulfosuccinate is a disodium salt of a substituted ethanolamide half ester of sulfosuccinic acid.

Class: Sulfosuccinates, Sulfosuccinamates

Function: Surfactants—Cleansing Agent, Foam Booster

Found in: Shampoos, Conditioners, Miscellaneous

Other Names: Disodium Monolauramido MEA-Sulfosuccinate

Disodium Laureth Sulfosuccinate (dy-SOH-dee-um LOHR-eth SUL-foh-sook-in-ayt)

Definition: Disodium laureth sulfosuccinate is the disodium salt of an ethoxylated lauryl alcohol half ester of sulfosuccinic acid with an ethoxylation value between 1 and 4.

Class: Sulfosuccinates, Sulfosuccinamates

Function: Surfactants—Cleansing Agent, Foam Booster
Found in: Shampoos, Conditioners, Miscellaneous
Other Names: Disodium Monolaureth Sulfosuccinate

Disodium Lauroamphodipropionate (dy-SOH-dee-um LOHR-oh-amp-foh-dy-prohp-ee-oh-nayt)

Definition: Disodium lauroamphodipropionate is an amphoteric surfactant.
Class: Alkylamido Alkylamines
Function: Surfactants—Cleansing Agent, Foam Booster, Conditioner
Found in: Shampoos, Conditioners, Miscellaneous
Other Names: Lauroamphodipropionate, Lauroamphocarboxypropionate

Disodium Lauryl Sulfosuccinate (dy-SOH-dee-um LOHR-uhl SUL-foh-sook-in-ayt)

Definition: Disodium lauryl sulfosuccinate is a disodium salt of a lauryl alcohol half ester of sulfosuccinic acid.
Class: Sulfosuccinates, Sulfosuccinamates
Function: Surfactants—Cleansing Agent, Foam Booster
Found in: Shampoos, Miscellaneous
Other Names: Disodium Monolauryl Sulfosuccinate

Disodium Oleamido PEG-2 Sulfosuccinate (dy-SOH-dee-um OH-lee-uh-my-doh SUL-foh-sook-in-ayt)

Definition: Disodium oleamido PEF-2-sulfosuccinate is the disodium salt of the monooleyl amide of the PEG-2 half ester of sulfosuccinic acid.
Class: Sulfosuccinates, Sulfosuccinamates
Function: Surfactants—Cleansing Agent, Foam Booster
Found in: Shampoos, Conditioners, Miscellaneous
Other Names: Oleoyl Disodium Sulfosuccinoyl Amide

Disodium Phosphate (dy-SOH-dee-um FAHS-fayt)

Definition: Disodium phosphate is an inorganic salt used to adjust pH.

Class: Inorganic Salts, Phosphorus Compounds
Function: pH Adjusters
Found in: Shampoos, Conditioners, Hair Dyes, Hair Colorants, Permanent Waves, Miscellaneous
Other Names: Dibasic Sodium Phosphate, Disodium Hydrogen Phosphate

D

Disodium Ricinoleamido MEA-Sulfosuccinate (dy-SOH-dee-um RIK-in-oh-lee-uh-my-doh SUL-foh-sook-in-ayt)
Definition: Disodium ricinoleamido MEA-sulfosuccinate is a disodium salt of a substituted ethanolamide half ester of sulfosuccinic acid.
Class: Sulfosuccinates and Sulfosuccinamates
Function: Surfactants—Cleansing Agent, Foam Booster
Found in: Shampoos, Baby Shampoos
Other Names: Disodium Monoricinoleamido MEA-Sulfosuccinate

Disodium Tallowamphodiacetate (dy-SOH-dee-um tal-oh-am-foh-dy-AS-uh-tayt)
Definition: Disodium tallowamphodiacetate is an amphoteric surfactant derived from tallow.
Class: Alkylamido Alkylamines
Function: Surfactants—Cleansing Agent, Foam Booster, Conditioner
Found in: Shampoos, Conditioners, Miscellaneous
Other Names: None Available

Disperse Blue 1 (DIS-purs BLOO)
Definition: Disperse blue 1 is an organic anthraquinone hair colorant.
Class: Hair Colorant
Function: Hair Colorant
Found in: Hair Dyes, Hair Colorants
Other Names: Solvent Blue 18

Distearyldimonium Chloride (dy-STEER-al-dy-MOH-nee-um KHLOR-yd)

Definition: Distearyldimonium chloride is a quaternary ammonium salt.

Class: Quaternary Ammonium Compounds

Function: Conditioners—Antistatic

Found in: Shampoos, Conditioners, Hairsprays, Setting Lotions, Miscellaneous

Other Names: Quaternium 5, Distearyl Dimethyl Ammonium Chloride

Ditallowdimonium Chloride (dy-tal-oh-DY-moh-nee-um KHLOR-eyed)

Definition: Ditallowdimonium chloride is a quaternary ammonium salt derived from tallow.

Class: Quaternary Ammonium Compounds

Function: Conditioners—Antistatic

Found in: Conditioners, Hairsprays, Aerosol Hairsprays, Miscellaneous

Other Names: Quaternium-48, Dimethyl Ditallow Ammonium Chloride

Dithiothreitol (dy-THY-oh-three-eh-tohl)

Definition: Dithiothreitol is an organic thio compound.

Class: Thio Compounds

Function: Hair Waving and Straightening—Reducing Agent

Found in: Permanent Waves, Hair Straighteners

Other Names: Dimercaptobutanediol, Cleland's Reagent

DMDM Hydantoin (hy-DAN-shun)

Definition: DMDM hydantoin is an organic compound used as a broad-spectrum antimicrobial that is effective against bacteria, fungi, and yeasts. Its effectiveness is increased with the use of parabens. Although it is considered to be a possible formaldehyde donor, it has not been established that DMDM hydantoin can release formaldehyde in hair care products.

Class: Amides, Heterocyclic Compounds
Function: Preservative
Found in: Shampoos, Conditioners, Hairsprays, Setting Lotions, Permanent Waves, Hair Straighteners, Hair Dyes, Hair Colorants, Miscellaneous
Other Names: DMDMH, N,N-Dimethylol-5,5-Dimethylhydantoin

DNA

Definition: DNA is a polynucleotide found mainly in the chromosomes of cell nuclei. When hydrolyzed, DNA yields guanine, adenine, cytosine, and thymine N-2-deoxyribosides.
Class: Biological Polymers
Function: Conditioner
Found in: Shampoos, Conditioners, Miscellaneous
Other Names: Deoxyribonucleic Acid

Dodecylbenzene Sulfonic Acid (doh-dek-ul-BEN-zeen SUL-fohn-ik AS-ud)

Definition: Dodecylbenzene sulfonic acid is a substituted aromatic acid surfactant. It is a powerful detergent, but is known to be a primary irritant that is drying to the skin.
Class: Alkyl Aryl Sulfonates
Function: Surfactants—Cleansing Agent
Found in: Shampoos
Other Names: LAS Acid, Linear Alkylbenzene Sulfonate

Dodoxynol-6 (doh-DAHKS-uh-nohl)

Definition: Dodoxynol-6 is an ethoxylated alkyl phenol surfactant with an average ethoxylation value of 6.
Class: Alkoxylated Alcohols
Function: Surfactants—Emulsifying Agent
Found in: Shampoos, Conditioners, Miscellaneous
Other Names: PEG-6 Dodecyl Phenyl Ether

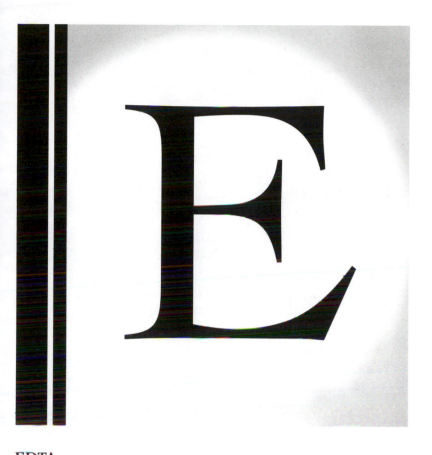

EDTA

Definition: EDTA is a substituted diamine. It is frequently used in the form of a partly neutralized salt (Disodium EDTA). EDTA is used as a chelating agent to prevent unwanted reactions with the trace metals that are inevitably present in hair care products. It stabilizes product color and keeps clear products clear. As an antioxidant, it prevents unsaturated oils from becoming rancid. It also enhances the antibacterial activity of parabens and imidazolidinyl urea.

Class: Alkyl-Substituted Amino Acids

Function: Chelating Agent, Preservative

Found in: Shampoos, Conditioners, Setting Lotions, Hair Dyes, Hair Colorants, Permanent Waves, Miscellaneous

Other Names: Edetic Acid, Ethylene Diamine Tetra Acetic Acid

Elastin (ee-LAS-tin)

Definition: Elastin is a fibrous protein found in the connective tissue of animals.

Class: Proteins

Function: Conditioner

Found in: Shampoos, Conditioners, Miscellaneous

Other Names: None Available

Equisetum Arvense Extract (eh-KWEE-she-tum AR-vens EKS-tract)

Definition: Equisetum arvense extract is an extract of the whole herb *Equisetum arvense* (horsetail).

Class: Biological

Function: Conditioner

Found in: Shampoos, Conditioners, Permanent Waves, Miscellaneous

Other Names: Horsetail Extract

Ergocalciferol (ur-go-kal-SIF-ur-awl)

Definition: Ergocalciferol is a synthetic vitamin D, prepared by UV irradiation of ergosterol. It is a sterol and may have some conditioning effect if used in sufficient quantity.

Class: Alcohols, Sterols

Function: Conditioners—Moisturizer

Found in: Shampoos, Conditioners, Setting Lotions, Miscellaneous

Other Names: Calciferol, Viosterol, Vitamin D, Vitamin D-12

Ethanolamine (eth-an-awl-AM-een)

Definition: Ethanolamine is a monoamine, organic alkali. It is used as an alkalizing agent and has become popular as an ammonia substitute in haircolorants and permanent waves.

Class: Alkanolamines

Function: pH adjuster

Found in: Hair Dyes, Hair Colorants, Permanent Waves, Hair Straighteners, Miscellaneous

Other Names: Monoethanolamine, 2-Aminoethanol, 2-Hydroxyethylamine

E

Ethanolamine Dithioglycolate (eth-an-awl-AM-een dy-thy-oh-GLY-kuh-layt)

Definition: Ethanolamine dithioglycolate is the salt of thioglycolic acid and ethanolamine.

Class: Organic Salts, Thio Compounds

Function: Hair Waving and Straightening — Reducing Agent, Depilatory

Found in: Permanent Waves, Hair Straighteners, Depilatories

Other Names: Ethanolamine Thioglycolate, Monoethanolamine Thioglycolate

Ethoxydiglycol (eth-ahks-ee-di-GLY-kawl)

Definition: Ethoxydiglycol is an ether alcohol similar to propylene glycol and butylene glycol that is used as a solvent to dissolve botanical extracts. Although it has humectant properties, it is more irritating than similar humectants and is normally used as a solvent.

Class: Alcohols, Ethers

Function: Solvent

Found in: Shampoos, Conditioners, Hairsprays, Setting Lotions, Hair Dyes, Hair Colorants, Bleaches, Miscellaneous

Other Names: Diethylene Glycol Monoethyl Ether

Ethoxyethanol (eth-ahks-ee-ETH-an-awl)

Definition: Ethoxyethanol is an ether alcohol.

Class: Alcohols, Ethers

Function: Solvent

Found in: Shampoos
Other Names: Ethylene Glycol Monoethyl Ether

4-Ethoxy-m-phenylenediamine Sulfate (eth-AHKS-ee fen-ul-een-dy-AM-een SUL-fayt)

Definition: 4-Ethoxy-m-phenylenediamine sulfate is a substituted aromatic amine salt used as a hair colorant.
Class: Amines
Function: Hair Colorant
Found in: Hair Dyes, Hair Colorants
Other Names: 4-ethoxy-1,3-Benzenediamine Sulfate

Ethylcellulose (eth-ul-SEL-u-lohs)

Definition: Ethylcellulose is an ethyl ether of cellulose.
Class: Carbohydrates, Ethers
Function: Thickener
Found in: Shampoos, Conditioners, Miscellaneous
Other Names: Cellulose Ethyl Ether

Ethyl Ester of PVM/MA Copolymer (ETH-ul ES-ter KOH-pahl-uh-mur)

Definition: Ethyl ester of PVM/MA copolymer is a polymer consisting of the partial ethyl ester of the polycarboxylic resin formed from vinyl methyl ether and maleic anhydride.
Class: Esters, Synthetic Polymers
Function: Hair Fixative, Film Former
Found in: Hairsprays, Aerosol Hairsprays, Setting Lotions
Other Names: Vinyl Methyl Ether Ethyl Maleate Copolymer

Ethyl Hexanediol (ETH-ul HEKS-ayn-dy-awl)

Definition: Ethyl hexanediol is an aliphatic alcohol that is a good solvent and emollient, resembling glycerol in its lubricating ability. It is also a well-known insect repellent.
Class: Alcohol
Function: Solvent

Found in: Shampoos, Conditioners, Miscellaneous
Other Names: Octylene Glycol, Ethohexadiol

Ethylhexyl Dimethyl PABA (ETH-ul-heks-ul dy-METH-ul PAH-bah)

Definition: Ethylhexyl dimethyl PABA is the ester of 2-ethyl-hexyl alcohol and dimethyl p-aminobenzoic acid that is used as a sunscreen. When used as an active drug ingredient, the established name is Padimate O.

Class: PABA Derivatives

Function: Sunscreen, UV light Absorber

Found in: Shampoos, Conditioners, Hairsprays, Setting Lotions, Suntan Lotions, Miscellaneous

Other Names: Padimate O, Octyl Dimethyl PABA

Ethylhexyl Methoxycinnamate (ETH-ul-heks-ul meth-ahks-ee-SIN-uh-mayt)

Definition: Ethylhexyl methoxycinnamate is the ester of 2-ethylhexyl alcohol and methoxycinnamic acid. When used as an active drug ingredient, the established name is Octinoxate.

Class: Esters

Function: Sunscreen, UV light Absorber

Found in: Shampoos, Conditioners, Hairsprays, Setting Lotions, Suntan Lotions, Miscellaneous

Other Names: Octinoxate, Octyl Methoxycinnamate

Ethylhexyl Salicylate (ETH-ul-heks-ul sal-uh-SY-layt)

Definition: Ethylhexyl salicylate is an ester of 2-ethylhexyl alcohol and salicylic acid. When used as an active drug ingredient, the established name is Octisalate.

Class: Esters, Phenols

Function: Sunscreen, UV light Absorber

Found in: Shampoos, Conditioners, Hairsprays, Setting Lotions, Suntan Lotions, Miscellaneous

Other Names: Octisalate, Octyl Salicylate

E

Ethyl Linoleate (ETH-ul LIN-oh-lee-ayt)

Definition: Ethyl linoleate is an ester of ethyl alcohol and linoleic acid.

Class: Esters

Function: Conditioners—Moisturizer

Found in: Hair Bleaches, Miscellaneous

Other Names: Linoleic Acid Ethyl Ester

Ethyl Paraben (ETH-ul PAR-uh-ben)

Definition: Ethyl paraben is the ester of ethyl alcohol and p-hydroxybenzoic acid.

Class: Esters, Phenols

Function: Preservative

Found in: Shampoos, Conditioners, Hairsprays, Setting Lotions, Hair Dyes, Hair Colorants, Miscellaneous

Other Names: Ethyl 4-Hydroxybenzoate, Parahydroxybenzoate ester

Ethyl Stearate (ETH-ul STEER-ayt)

Definition: Ethyl stearate is an ester of ethyl alcohol and stearic acid.

Class: Esters

Function: Conditioners—Moisturizer

Found in: Shampoos, Conditioners, Miscellaneous

Other Names: Ethyl Octadecanoate

Ext. Violet 2 (VY-oh-let)

Definition: Ext. violet 2 is an anthraquinone colorant.

Class: Colorant

Function: Colorant

Found in: Shampoos, Conditioners, Hairsprays, Setting Lotions, Hair Dyes, Hair Colorants, Hair Bleaches, Miscellaneous

Other Names: Ext. D&C Violet No. 2, Alizarine Violet, Alizarin Irisol R

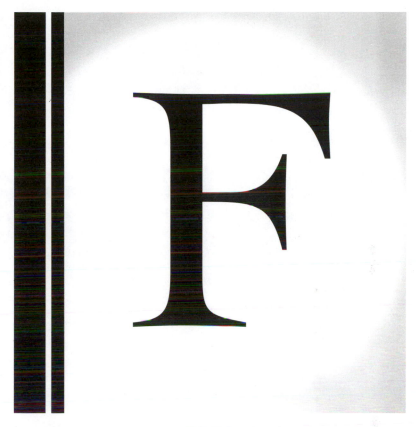

Fast Green FCF (FAST GREEN)

Definition: Fast green FCF is a triphenylmethane colorant.

Class: Colorant

Function: Colorant

Found in: Shampoos, Conditioners, Hairsprays, Setting Lotions, Hair Dyes, Hair Colorants, Miscellaneous

Other Names: Food Green 3, Green No. 3, Japan Green 3

Formaldehyde (for-MAL-duh hyd)

Definition: Although formaldehyde is an effective, broadspectrum fungicide and bactericide, there are concerns about its safety in cosmetics. It is extremely irritating, toxic, and a known allergen.

Class: Aldehydes

Function: Preservative

Found in: Shampoos, Conditioners, Hairsprays, Setting Lotions, Hair Dyes, Hair Colorants, Miscellaneous

Other Names: Formalin, Formic Aldehyde, Merthaldehyde, Methanal, Methyl Aldehyde, Oxomethane, Oxymethylene

F

Fragrance (FRAY-grentz)

Definition: Fragrance is a term for ingredient labeling used to identify a product that contains a material or a combination of materials added to produce or to mask a particular odor. Although the product must list a fragrance, the ingredients of the fragrance do not need to be listed.

Class: Fragrance

Function: Fragrance

Found in: Shampoos, Conditioners, Hairsprays, Setting Lotions, Hair Dyes, Hair Colorants, Permanent Waves, Hair Straighteners, Miscellaneous

Other Names: None Available

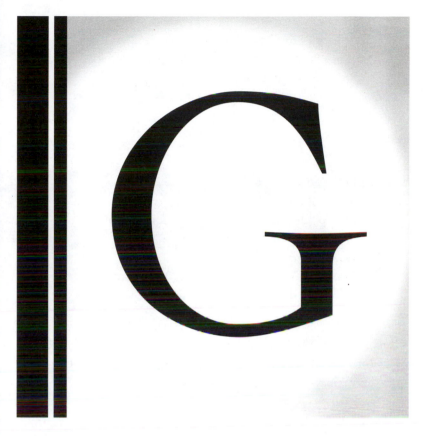

Gelatin (JEL-ut-un)

Definition: Gelatin is obtained by the partial hydrolysis of collagen derived from the skin, tendons, ligaments, and bones of animals. Although it is a protein, it is not effective as a conditioner due to its high molecular weight.

Class: Gums, Colloids, Proteins

Function: Thickener

Found in: Shampoos, Conditioners, Miscellaneous

Other Names: Gelatine, Gelatin Velvatex

Glucose Glutamate (GLOO-kohs GLOO-tuh-mayt)

Definition: Glucose glutamate is formed from a saccharide (glucose) and an amino acid (glutamic acid), which are two components of the natural moisturizing factor of the skin. It is a humectant and conditioner that leaves a film that makes hair smoother and more manageable, increases shine, and improves wet combing.

Class: Amino Acids, Carbohydrates, Esters
Function: Conditioners—Moisturizer
Found in: Shampoos, Conditioners, Miscellaneous
Other Names: None Available

G

Glutaral (GLOO-tah-rahl)

Definition: Glutaral is a broad-spectrum antimicrobial, which is more potent but less irritating than formaldehyde.
Class: Aldehydes
Function: Preservative
Found in: Shampoos, Conditioners, Miscellaneous
Other Names: Glutaraldehyde, Glutaric Dialdehyde, Pentanedial

Glycereth-26 (GLIS-ur-eth)

Definition: Glycereth-26 is the polyethylene glycol ether of glycerin with an average ethoxylation value of 26.
Class: Alkoxylated Alcohols
Function: Conditioners—Moisturizer
Found in: Shampoos, Conditioners, Hair Dyes, Hair Colorants, Miscellaneous
Other Names: PEG-26 Glyceryl Ether, Polyethylene Glycol (26) Glyceryl Ether

Glycerin (GLIS-ur-in)

Definition: Glycerin is a polyhydric alcohol that is a normal by-product of human metabolism. It is nontoxic and nonirritating to skin, and is not known to produce allergic skin reactions. The correct name for pure glycerin is glycerol. Glycerin was first produced by the hydrolysis of fats during the manufacture of soaps, but it can also be produced synthetically from propylene.

Glycerin is a humectant that moistens and softens hair and skin. These same humectant properties also help prevent products such as toothpaste from drying out when the cap is left off the tube.

Class: Polyols

Function: Conditioners — Moisturizer

Found in: Shampoos, Conditioners, Hairsprays, Setting Lotions, Hair Dyes, Hair Colorants, Permanent Waves, Hair Straighteners, Miscellaneous

Other Names: Glycerol, Glycyl Alcohol, 1,2,3-Propanetriol, 1,2,3-Trihydroxypropane

G

Glyceryl Laurate (GLIS-ur-ul LOR-ayt)

Definition: Glyceryl laurate is the monoester of glycerin and lauric acid.

Class: Glyceryl Esters

Function: Surfactants — Emulsifying Agent

Found in: Shampoos, Setting Lotions, Permanent Waves, Miscellaneous

Other Names: Glyceryl Monolaurate, 1-Monododecanoyl-glycerol, 1-Monolaurin

Glyceryl Stearate (GLIS-ur-ul STEER-ayt)

Definition: Glyceryl stearate is the monoester of glycerin and stearic acid.

Class: Glyceryl Esters

Function: Surfactants — Emulsifying Agent, Conditioner

Found in: Shampoos, Conditioners, Hairsprays, Setting Lotions, Hair Dyes, Hair Colorants, Permanent Waves, Hair Straighteners, Miscellaneous

Other Names: Glycerin 1-Stearate, Glyceryl Monostearate, Glycerol 1-Stearate, Monostearin

Glycine (GLY-seen)

Definition: Glycine is an amino acid often used to adjust the pH of the finished product. Amino acids are also good moisturizers and are a major component of the natural moisturizing factor (NMF) of the skin.

Class: Amino Acids

Function: pH Adjusters, Conditioners—Moisturizer

Found in: Shampoos, Conditioners, Miscellaneous

Other Names: Aminoacetic Acid, Aminoethanoic Acid, Glycocoll

G Glycol (GLY-kawl)

Definition: Glycol is an aliphatic diol.

Class: Alcohols

Function: Fragrance, Solvent, Humectant

Found in: Permanent Waves

Other Names: 1,2 Ethanediol, Ethylene Glycol, 2-Hydroxyethanol

Glycol Distearate (GLY-kawl dy-STEER-ayt)

Definition: Glycol distearate is a diester of ethylene glycol and stearic acid. It is most often used as a conditioner or coemulsifier. It is practically nontoxic and nonirritating.

Class: Esters

Function: Conditioners—Moisturizer, Coemulsifier, Pearling Agent

Found in: Shampoos, Conditioners, Hair Dyes, Hair Colorants, Permanent Waves, Miscellaneous

Other Names: Ethylene Glycol Distearate, Ethylene Dioctadecanoate

Glycolic Acid (gly-KAWL-ik AS-ud)

Definition: Glycolic acid occurs naturally in small amounts, but is usually synthesized either by hydrolysis of chloracetic acid or oxidation of ethylene glycol. It is safer than mineral acids and has no odor.

Class: Carboxylic Acids

Function: pH Adjuster

Found in: Shampoos, Conditioners, Miscellaneous

Other Names: Hydroxyacetic Acid, Hydroxyethanoic Acid

Glycol Stearate (GLY-kawl STEER-ayt)

Definition: Glycol stearate is an ester of ethylene glycol and stearic acid. It is most often used as a pearling agent. It is practically nontoxic and nonirritating.

Class: Esters

Function: Conditioners—Moisturizer, Coemulsifier, Pearling Agent

Found in: Shampoos, Conditioners, Hair Dyes, Hair Colorants, Miscellaneous

Other Names: Ethylene Glycol Monostearate, Glycol Monostearate

Green 5 (GREEN)

Definition: Green 5 is an anthraquinone colorant.

Class: Colorants

Function: Colorant

Found in: Shampoos, Conditioners, Hair Dyes, Hair Colorants, Miscellaneous

Other Names: D&C Green No. 5

Guanidine Carbonate (GWAN-uh-deen KAR-bon-ayt)

Definition: Guanidine carbonate is an organic alkali. It is used in two-part, "no lye," over-the-counter hair relaxer kits. Mixing guanidine carbonate with calcium hydroxide immediately before use forms guanidine hydroxide, which is the relaxer's active ingredient.

Class: Organic Salts

Function: Hair Straightening—Hydroxide Relaxers

Found in: Hair Straighteners

Other Names: Diguanidinium Carbonate

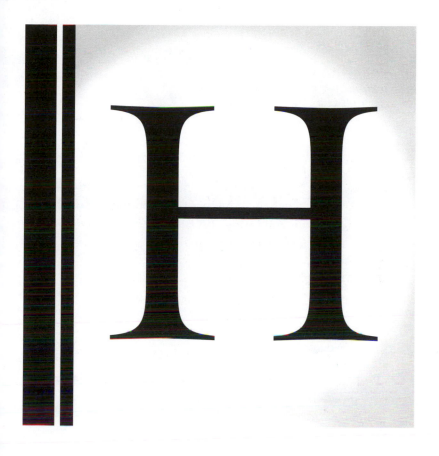

Hamamelis Virginiana (Witch Hazel) Extract (HAM-uh-mel-is vur-JIN-ee-ahn-uh)

Definition: Hamamelis virginiana (witch hazel) extract is an extract of the bark, leaves, and twigs of the witch hazel *Hamamelis virginiana*.

Class: Biological Products

Function: Natural Ingredients

Found in: Shampoos, Conditioners, Hairsprays, Miscellaneous

Other Names: Hamamelis Extract, Witch Hazel Extract

HC Orange No. 1 (OR-anj)

Definition: HC orange No. 1 is an organic hair colorant.
Class: Hair Colorants
Function: Hair Colorant
Found in: Hair Dyes, Hair Colorants
Other Names: 2-Nitro-4-Hydroxydiphenylamine

Hectorite (HEK-tow-ryt)

Definition: Hectorite is one of the montmorillonite minerals that are the principal constituents of bentonite clay. It is used to thicken emulsions and suspend heavy compounds. It lubricates and gives hair a smooth feel.
Class: Inorganics
Function: Thickener, Conditioners—Moisturizer
Found in: Shampoos, Conditioners, Miscellaneous
Other Names: None Available

Henna (HEN-uh)

Definition: Henna is the natural material derived from the dried powdered leaves of the shrub *Lawsonia inermis*. It contains the coloring agent lawsone, which is 2-hydroxy-1,4-naphthoquinone. It is relatively nontoxic.
Class: Hair Colorants
Function: Hair Colorant
Found in: Shampoos, Conditioners, Hair Dyes, Hair Colorants
Other Names: Lawsonia Alba, Camphire

Hexylene Glycol (HEKS-uh-leen GLY-kawl)

Definition: Hexylene glycol is an aliphatic alcohol.
Class: Alcohols
Function: Solvent, Fragrance
Found in: Shampoos, Conditioners, Hair Dyes, Hair Colorants, Miscellaneous
Other Names: 2-Methyl-2,4-Pentanediol

Homosalate (hoh-moh-SAH-layt)
Definition: Homosalate is a substituted phenolic compound.
Class: Esters, Phenols
Function: Sunscreen, UV Light Absorber
Found in: Suntan Products and Lotions
Other Names: Homomenthyl Salicylate

Hydrated Silica (HY-drah-ted SIL-uh-kah)
Definition: Hydrated silica is an inorganic oxide.
Class: Inorganics
Function: Thickener, Conditioners — Moisturizer
Found in: Hair Bleaches
Other Names: Hydrosilicic Acid, Silica Gel, Silicic Acid
Hydrate

Hydrofluorocarbon 152A (hy-droh-FLOHR-oh-kar-bon)
Definition: Hydrofluorocarbon 152A is a halocarbon used as
a propellant in aerosol hairsprays. This propellant is envi-
ronmentally friendly and is used in place of chlorofluoro-
carbons (CFCs).
Class: Halogen Compounds
Function: Propellant
Found in: Aerosol Hairsprays
Other Names: Ethylidene Fluoride, Fluorocarbon 152a,
HFC 152a

Hydrogenated Jojoba Oil (HY-druh-jen-ayt-ud hoh-HOH-ba OIL)
Definition: Hydrogenated jojoba oil is the end product of the
hydrogenation of *Simmondsia chinensis* (jojoba) oil.
Class: Waxes
Function: Conditioners — Moisturizer
Found in: Shampoos, Conditioners, Hairsprays, Hair Dyes,
Hair Colorants, Miscellaneous
Other Names: None Available

H

Hydrogenated Polydecene (HY-druh-jen-ayt-ud pahl-ee-DEK-een)

Definition: Hydrogenated polydecene is the end product of the hydrogenation of polydecene.

Class: Synthetic Polymers

Function: Conditioners — Moisturizer

Found in: Shampoos

Other Names: 1-Decene Homopolymer hydrogenated

Hydrogenated Starch Hydrolysate (HY-druh-jen-ayt-ud STARCH HY-droh-ly-sayt)

Definition: Hydrogenated starch hydrolysate is a carbohydrate produced by the controlled hydrogenation of corn syrup.

Class: Carbohydrates

Function: Conditioners — Humectant

Found in: Shampoos

Other Names: Hydrogenated Corn Syrup

Hydrogenated Tallowtrimonium Chloride (HY-druh-jen-ayt-ud tal-oh-try-MOH-nee-um KLOR-eyed)

Definition: Hydrogenated tallowtrimonium chloride is a quaternary ammonium salt produced from animal tallow. Hydrogenated tallow derivatives are similar to stearic acid compounds and contain stearic, oleic, and palmitic fatty acids. Hydrogenated tallowtrimonium chloride is used as a cationic emulsifying agent, and is also a substantive conditioning agent that imparts softness and manageability to hair. It is corrosive to skin and eyes due to its cationic nature.

Class: Quaternary Ammonium Compounds

Function: Conditioners — Antistatic

Found in: Shampoos, Conditioners, Miscellaneous

Other Names: Hydrogenated Tallow Alkyl Trimethyl Chloride

Hydrogenated Vegetable Oil (HY-druh-jen-ayt-ud VEJ-uh-tah-bul OYL)

Definition: Hydrogenated vegetable oil is produced by the controlled hydrogenation of vegetable oil.

Class: Fats and Oils
Function: Conditioners — Moisturizer, Thickener
Found in: Shampoos, Conditioners, Miscellaneous
Other Names: None Available

Hydrogen Peroxide (HY-druh-jen pur-AHK-syd)

Definition: Hydrogen peroxide (H_2O_2) is an inorganic oxidizing agent. It can be thought of as water with an "extra" oxygen. Diluted solutions of hydrogen peroxide are used in haircoloring and permanent waving. The term "volume" indicates the concentration and strength of solutions of hydrogen peroxide. Higher volumes of hydrogen peroxide contain higher percentages, which make them stronger because they are more concentrated.

The developer used with most haircolorants is between 10 volume (3 percent), to 20 volume (6 percent) hydrogen peroxide. Hair lighteners and bleaches may contain higher concentrations of hydrogen peroxide that are considerably stronger. Hydrogen peroxide is also used in concentrations up to 10 volume (3 percent) in permanent waving neutralizers.

Class: Inorganics
Function: Oxidizers
Found in: Hair Dyes, Hair Colorants, Bleaches, Hair Lighteners, Permanent Wave Neutralizers
Other Names: Hydrogen Dioxide

Hydrolyzed Collagen (HY-droh-lyzed KAHL-uh-jen)

Definition: Hydrolyzed collagen is the hydrolysate of animal collagen. Hydrolysis by acid, enzyme, or other methods splits the collagen proteins, breaking them down into their smaller component parts.

Class: Protein Derivatives
Function: Conditioners — Humectant

Found in: Shampoos, Conditioners, Hairsprays, Setting Lotions, Hair Dyes, Hair Colorants, Permanent Waves, Hair Straighteners, Miscellaneous

Other Names: Collagen Hydrolysate, Hydrolyzed Animal Protein

Hydrolyzed Elastin (HY-droh-lyzed ee-LAS-tin)

Definition: Hydrolyzed elastin is the hydrolysate of elastin derived by acid, enzyme, or other method of hydrolysis. The amino acid composition of elastin differs significantly from that of collagen. It is an excellent moisturizer and film-forming agent used in conditioners to help repair chemically damaged hair to improve the feel, body, and wet combing.

Class: Protein Derivatives

Function: Conditioners — Humectant

Found in: Shampoos, Conditioners, Hairsprays, Setting Lotions, Hair Dyes, Hair Colorants, Miscellaneous

Other Names: Elastin Hydrolysate, Hydrolyzed Animal Elastin

Hydrolyzed Glycosaminoglycans (HY-droh-lyzed gly-kohs-uh-MEE-noh-gly-kans)

Definition: Hydrolyzed glycosaminoglycans is a mixture of polysaccharides derived from the hydrolysis of animal connective tissue, consisting chiefly of glucosamine and glucuronic acid.

Class: Carbohydrates

Function: Conditioners — Humectant

Found in: Shampoos, Conditioners, Hairsprays, Setting Lotions, Hair Dyes, Hair Colorants, Miscellaneous

Other Names: Hydrolyzed Mucopolysaccharides, Mucopolysaccharide Hydrolysate

Hydrolyzed Hair Keratin (HY-droh-lyzed HAYR KER-uh-tin)

Definition: Hydrolyzed hair keratin is the hydrolysate of human hair keratin derived by acid, enzyme, or other method of hydrolysis.

Class: Protein Derivatives
Function: Conditioners—Humectant
Found in: Shampoos, Conditioners, Hairsprays, Setting Lotions, Hair Dyes, Hair Colorants, Miscellaneous
Other Names: Hair Keratin Hydrolysate, Protein, Hydrolyzed Hair Keratin

Hydrolyzed Silk (HY-droh-lyzed SILK)

Definition: Hydrolyzed silk is the hydrolysate of silk protein derived by acid, enzyme, or other method of hydrolysis.
Class: Protein Derivatives
Function: Conditioners—Humectant
Found in: Shampoos, Conditioners, Hairsprays, Setting Lotions, Hair Dyes, Hair Colorants, Miscellaneous
Other Names: Silk Hydrolysate, Silk Protein

Hydrolyzed Vegetable Protein (HY-droh-lyzed VEJ-uh-tah-bul PROH-teen)

Definition: Hydrolyzed vegetable protein is the hydrolysate of vegetable protein derived from acid, enzyme, or other method of hydrolysis. Plants contain lower concentrations of protein than those found in animals. Vegetable proteins are often used as an alternative to animal proteins in products that are marketed as being manufactured from nonanimal ingredients.
Class: Protein Derivatives
Function: Conditioners—Humectant
Found in: Shampoos, Conditioners, Hairsprays, Setting Lotions, Hair Dyes, Hair Colorants, Miscellaneous
Other Names: Vegetable Protein Hydrolysate

Hydrolyzed Wheat Protein (HY-droh-lyzed WHEET PROH-teen)

Definition: Hydrolyzed wheat protein is the hydrolysate of wheat protein derived by acid, enzyme, or other method of hydrolysis.

Class: Protein Derivatives

Function: Conditioners—Humectant

Found in: Shampoos, Conditioners, Hairsprays, Setting Lotions, Hair Dyes, Hair Colorants, Miscellaneous

Other Names: Wheat Protein Hydrolysate

Hydroxyethylcellulose (hy-draks-ee-eth-ul-SEL-yoo-lohs)

Definition: Hydroxyethylcellulose is a modified cellulose polymer formed by the addition of ethylene oxide to cellulose. Various grades are available with different ratios of cellulose to ethylene oxide.

Class: Gums, Hydrophilic Colloids

Function: Thickener, Emulsion Stabilizer, Film Former

Found in: Shampoos, Conditioners, Hairsprays, Setting Lotions, Hair Dyes, Hair Colorants, Miscellaneous

Other Names: Cellulose Hydroxyethylate, H. E. Cellulose, Cellulose 2-Hydroxyethyl Ether

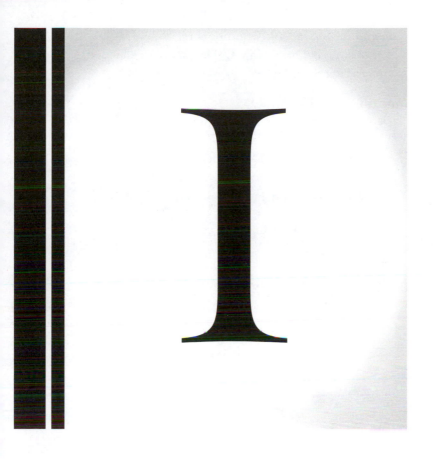

Imidazolidinyl Urea (im-id-AZ-oh-lid-in-ul YUR-ee-uh)

Definition: Imidazolidinyl urea is a heterocyclic urea with antimicrobial properties that is used as a preservative. It is considered nontoxic but can cause allergic reactions. Although it is a formaldehyde donor, formaldehyde-sensitive patients do not react to it. Diazolidinyl urea is a similar material that was developed as an improvement to imidazolidinyl urea.

Class: Amides, Heterocyclic Compounds

Function: Preservative

Found in: Shampoos, Conditioners, Hairsprays, Setting Lotions, Hair Dyes, Hair Colorants, Miscellaneous
Other Names: Imidurea

Inositol (in-AHS-uh-tahl)

Definition: Inositol is a cyclic polyol that is also known as meat sugar. Inositol occurs in all living cells and is a member of the vitamin B complex.
Class: Polyols
Function: Conditioners—Humectant
Found in: Shampoos, Conditioners, Miscellaneous
Other Names: Myoinosite, Phaseomannitol, Cyclohexanehexol

Iron Oxide (EYE-urn AHKS-eyed)

Definition: Iron oxide is an inorganic compound consisting of any one or combination of synthetically prepared iron oxides. Iron oxide is a range of pigments that varies in shade from yellow to red and black according to the chemical composition, method of manufacture, and blend used. Iron oxide is approved for use in animal foods and certain drugs, and is exempt from FDA certification.
Class: Color Additives
Function: Colorant
Found in: Shampoos, Conditioners, Miscellaneous
Other Names: Black Oxide of Iron, Brown Iron Oxide, Iron Oxide Red, Pigment Black 11, Pigment Brown 6, Pigment Red 101, Pigment Yellow 42, Red Iron Oxide, Yellow Iron Oxide

Isobutane (EYE-soh-BYOOT-ayn)

Definition: Isobutane is a hydrocarbon gas used in aerosol hairsprays as a propellant, and is usually used in combination with butane and propane. It is chemically inert, does not deplete the ozone, and is toxicologically safe, but it is inflammable.

Class: Hydrocarbons
Function: Propellant
Found in: Aerosol Hairsprays
Other Names: 1,1-Dimethylethane, 2-Methylpropane,
Trimethylmethane

Isoceteth-20 (eye-soh-SET-eth)

Definition: Isoceteth-20 is a polyethylene glycol ether of
isocetyl alcohol with an ethoxylation value of 20.
Class: Alkoxylated Alcohols
Function: Surfactants — Emulsifying Agent
Found in: Shampoos, Conditioners, Setting Lotions,
Miscellaneous
Other Names: PEG-20 Isocetyl Ether, Polyethylene Glycol
1000 Isocetyl Ether

Isodecane (eye-soh-DEK-ayn)

Definition: Isodecane is a branched chain aliphatic hydrocar-
bon with 12 carbons.
Class: Hydrocarbons
Function: Solvent
Found in: Aerosol Hairsprays
Other Names: 1,1-Dineopentylethylene, Isodecane (RIFM)

Isopropyl Alcohol (eye-soh-PROH-pal AL-kuh-hawl)

Definition: Isopropyl alcohol is an aliphatic alcohol with
many of the same properties as ethyl alcohol. Although it
is relatively nontoxic and nonirritating, it does have a
powerful drying effect on the skin. Isopropyl alcohol is
less flammable than ethyl alcohol, but has a stronger, less
pleasant odor. Isopropyl alcohol is used as a solvent for a
variety of ingredients that are not sufficiently water-
soluble. At high concentrations, it may be used as an
astringent and also has some antimicrobial properties.
Class: Alcohols
Function: Solvent

Found in: Shampoos, Conditioners, Hairsprays, Setting Lotions, Hair Dyes, Hair Colorants, Permanent Waves, Hair Straighteners

Other Names: Isopropanol, 2-Hydroxypropane, 1-Methylethanol, 2-Propanol

Isopropyl Myristate (eye-soh-PROH-pal MIR-uh-stayt)

Definition: Isopropyl myristate is the ester of isopropyl alcohol and myristic acid. It is nonirritating, nonallergenic, and harmless by ingestion. This is an excellent conditioner that provides outstanding spreading and penetration. It is often used to replace mineral oil because it is lighter and less greasy, and is used to replace vegetable oils because it is more stable and less likely to turn rancid. It is very similar to isopropyl palmitate.

Class: Esters

Function: Conditioners—Moisturizer

Found in: Shampoos, Conditioners, Hairsprays, Setting Lotions, Hair Dyes, Hair Colorants, Permanent Waves, Hair Straighteners

Other Names: Methyl Ethyl Myristate, Isopropyl Myristate, Isopropyl Tetradeconoate

Isostearic Acid (eye-soh-STEER-ik AS-ud)

Definition: Isostearic acid is a complex mixture of saturated branched chain fatty acids. It is relatively nontoxic and nonirritating with no significant eye irritation, but is known to be comedogenic.

Class: Fatty Acids

Function: Conditioners—Moisturizer, Emulsifying Agent

Found in: Shampoos, Conditioners, Miscellaneous

Other Names: Heptadecanoic Acid, Isooctadecanoic acid, 16-Methylheptadecanoic Acid

Isostearyl Alcohol (eye-soh-STEER-ul AL-kuh-hawl)

Definition: Isostearyl alcohol is a complex mixture of branched chain 18 carbon aliphatic alcohols produced by hydrogenation of isostearic acid.

Class: Fatty Alcohol

Function: Condtioners — Moisturizer, Emulsifier

Found in: Shampoos, Conditioners, Miscellaneous

Other Names: Isooctadecyl Alcohol, 16-Methyl-1-Heptadecanol

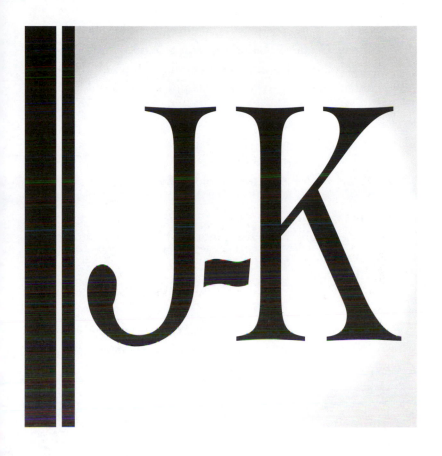

Jojoba Oil (hoh-HOH-ba OYL)

Definition: Jojoba oil is actually a liquid wax, not a true oil.
Jojoba oil the monohydric alcohol ester extracted from the
desert shrub *Simondsia chinesis*, which is native to the west-
ern United States. It is extremely popular because it is
considered to be a natural ingredient from a vegetable
source. Regardless of claims to the contrary, jojoba oil's
emollient and conditioning properties have not been

proven to be better than those of other vegetable or mineral oils. Crude jojoba oil contains a natural antioxidant that accounts for its excellent stability, although the refined material (bleached and stripped) is less stable to oxidation.

Class: Esters, Waxes
Function: Conditioners—Moisturizer
Found in: Shampoos, Conditioners, Miscellaneous
Other Names: Jojoba Esters, Jojoba Extract

Kaolin (KAY-uh-lin)

Definition: Kaolin is a native, inorganic, hydrated aluminum silicate.
Class: Inorganics
Function: Abrasive, Absorbant, Anticaking Agent, Bulking Agent
Found in: Shampoos, Conditioners, Hairsprays, Setting Lotions, Hair Dyes, Hair Colorants, Miscellaneous
Other Names: Bolus Alba, China Clay, Kaolite, Pigment White 19

Keratin Amino Acids (KAIR-uh-tin a-MEE-no AS-uds)

Definition: Keratin amino acids is the mixture of amino acids resulting from the hydrolysis (decomposition) of keratin proteins or polypeptides. The major amino acids in the mixture are glutamic acid, serine, proline, arginine, threonine, and aspartic acid. Keratin amino acids can be produced from human hair and wool as well as from animal horns and feathers. Different sources produce different blends of amino acids.

Keratin amino acids is a humectant conditioner used to maintain the hair's correct moisture balance, improve manageability and body, and add shine. This ingredient is extremely hydroscopic (attracts moisture) and is substantive to hair.

Keratin proteins are far too large to penetrate the hair. Hydrolysis of these proteins into keratin amino acids makes this ingredient more effective. Keratin amino acids penetrate hair due to its smaller molecular size (*see* Protein).

Class: Amino Acids

Function: Conditioners—Humectant, Film Former, Miscellaneous

Found in: Shampoos, Conditioners, Hairsprays, Setting Lotions, Hair Dyes, Hair Colorants, Miscellaneous

Other Names: Animal Keratin Amino Acids

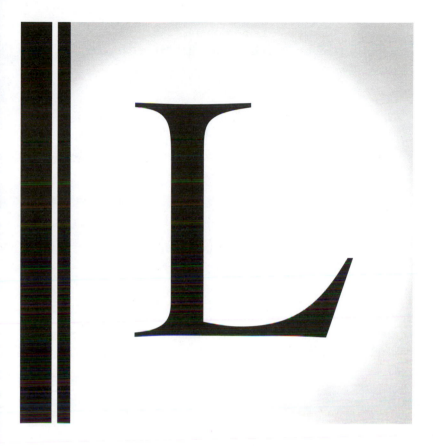

Lactic Acid (LAK-tik AS-ud)

Definition: Lactic acid is an organic hydroxy acid that naturally occurs in sour milk, formed by the action of *Streptococcus lactis* fermenting lactose. It is commercially prepared by the fermentation of carbohydrates. Lactic acid makes skin more pliable and is a component of the skin's natural moisturizing factor. It is frequently used to adjust the pH of hair care products because it also functions as a conditioner and humectant that increases the moisture content of hair.

Class: Carboxylic Acids

Function: Conditioners—Humectant, pH Adjuster

Found in: Shampoos, Conditioners, Hairsprays, Setting Lotions, Hair Dyes, Hair Colorants, Miscellaneous
Other Names: Alpha-Hydroxypropanoic Acid

Lactose (LAK-tohs)

Definition: Lactose, commonly called milk sugar, is a disaccharide obtained from the whey found in milk. It is unlikely to have any significant conditioning effects and is used primarily because of its appeal as a natural ingredient.
Class: Carbohydrate
Function: Conditioners—Miscellaneous
Found in: Shampoos, Conditioners, Miscellaneous
Other Names: Milk Sugar, Saccharum Lactin

Laneth 16 (LAN-eth)

Definition: Laneth-16 is a blend of ethoxylates prepared from lanolin alcohol. It is the polyethylene glycol ether of lanolin alcohol with an average ethoxylation value of 16. Laneth-16 is used as a nonionic emulsifier and provides some conditioning properties.
Class: Alkoxylated Alcohols, Lanolin and Lanolin Derivatives
Function: Surfactants—Emulsifying Agent
Found in: Shampoos, Conditioners, Miscellaneous
Other Names: PEG-16 Lanolin Ether, Polyoxyethylene Lanolin Ether

Lanolin (LAN-ul-un)

Definition: Lanolin is a complex mixture of esters and polyesters of high molecular weight, fatty acids, and alcohols obtained by refining wool grease, the secretion of the sebaceous glands of sheep. Lanolin is used as an emollient and conditioner, and forms an occlusive film on skin to prevent water loss.
Class: Lanolin and Lanolin Derivatives

Function: Conditioners — Moisturizer

Found in: Shampoos, Conditioners, Hairsprays, Setting Lotions, Hair Dyes, Hair Colorants, Permanent Waves, Hair Straighteners, Miscellaneous

Other Names: Anhydrous Lanolin, Wool Fat, Wool Wax

Lanolin Alcohol (LAN-ul-un AL-kuh-hawl)

Definition: Lanolin alcohol is a mixture of the organic fatty alcohols obtained from the hydrolysis of lanolin.

Class: Alcohols, Lanolin and Lanolin Derivatives

Function: Conditioners — Moisturizer, Thickener

Found in: Shampoos, Conditioners, Hairsprays, Setting Lotions, Hair Dyes, Hair Colorants, Permanent Waves, Hair Straighteners, Miscellaneous

Other Names: Wool Wax Alcohol

Lauramide DEA (LOR-uh-myd DEA)

Definition: Lauramide DEA is a mixture of ethanolamides of lauric acid. It is very effective as a foam booster and thickener when used with the anionic sulfate surfactants used in most shampoos.

Class: Alkanolamides

Function: Surfactants — Foam Booster, Thickener

Found in: Shampoos, Conditioners, Body Washes, Bubble Baths, Miscellaneous

Other Names: Lauric Acid Diethanolamide

Lauramidopropyl Betaine (LOR-uh-myd-oh-pro-pil BEE-tayn)

Definition: Lauramidopropyl betaine is a zwitterion that acts as a pseudoamphoteric surfactant. It is an extremely mild cleanser and foaming agent that is nonirritating to skin and eyes, and is often used in baby shampoos.

Class: Betaines

Function: Surfactants — Foam Booster, Cleanser, Conditioner, Thickener

Found in: Shampoos, Baby Shampoos, Conditioners, Bubble Baths, Body Cleansers, Miscellaneous

Other Names: Lauramidopropyl Dimethyl Glycine

Lauramine Oxide (LOR-uh-meen AHK-syd)

Definition: Lauramine oxide is a tertiary amine oxide surfactant used as a conditioner, foam booster, and thickener. It is cationic at an acid pH and a substantive conditioning agent with antistatic properties. It is nonionic at an alkaline pH and also used as a thickener. Amine oxides are very mild cleansers and have the ability to reduce the irritation of some other ingredients.

Class: Amine Oxides

Function: Surfactants—Cleansing Agent, Foam Booster, Conditioner, Thickener

Found in: Shampoos, Conditioners, Hairsprays, Setting Lotions, Hair Dyes, Hair Colorants, Miscellaneous

Other Names: Dodecyldimethylamine Oxide, Laurylamine Oxide

Laureth-4 (LOR-eth 4)

Definition: Laureth-4 is the polyethylene glycol ether of lauryl alcohol with an average ethoxylation value of 4. The number indicates the degree of ethoxylation (*see* ethoxylated surfactants). Higher ethoxylation produces ingredients with greater cleansing ability, but they foam less and have poor detergent qualities.

Class: Alkoxylated Alcohols

Function: Surfactants—Emulsifying Agent, Cleansing Agent, Foam Booster, Conditioner, Thickener

Found in: Shampoos, Conditioners, Hairsprays, Setting Lotions, Hair Dyes, Hair Colorants, Permanent Waves, Hair Straighteners, Miscellaneous

Other Names: PEG-4 Lauryl Ether, Polyethylene Glycol Ether, Polyoxyethylene (4) Lauryl Ether

Lauric Acid (LOR-ik AS-ud)

Definition: Lauric acid is a C12 carboxylic fatty acid usually produced from triglycerides such as coconut or palm kernel oil.

Class: Fatty Acids

Function: Surfactants—Cleansing Agent

Found in: Shampoos, Conditioners, Hairsprays, Setting Lotions, Hair Dyes, Hair Colorants, Miscellaneous

Other Names: n-Dodecanoic Acid, Dodecylic Acid

Lauryl Alcohol (LOR-ul AL-ku-hawl)

Definition: Lauryl alcohol is a mixture of the fatty alcohols dodecanol (C12) and tetradecanol (C14) produced from natural or synthetic sources. The natural source is usually coconut or palm kernel oil. Higher fatty alcohols such as cetyl alcohol, are usually preferred because they have less odor and produce a thicker cream.

Class: Fatty Alcohols

Function: Surfactants—Foam Booster, Conditioner, Thickener

Found in: Shampoos, Conditioners, Hairsprays, Setting Lotions, Hair Dyes, Hair Colorants, Permanent Waves, Hair Straighteners, Miscellaneous

Other Names: Didecyl Alcohol, 1-Dodecanol, 1-hydroxydodecane

Lauryl Betaine (LOR-ul BEE-tayn)

Definition: Lauryl betaine is a zwitterion similar to coco-betaine. Lauryl betaine is a pseudoamphoteric surfactant that is used as a mild cleansing agent, foam booster, conditioner, and thickener.

Class: Betaines

Function: Surfactants—Cleanser, Foam Booster, Conditioner, Thickener

Found in: Shampoos, Conditioners, Hair Dyes, Hair Colorants, Miscellaneous

Other Names: Dodecyldimethylbetaine, Lauryl Dimethyl Glycine

Lecithin (LES-uh-thin)

Definition: Lecithin is a naturally occurring mixture of the diglycerides of stearic, palmitic, and oleic acids linked to the choline ester of phosphoric acid. Lecithin is found in living plants and animals, and can be derived from eggs, soybeans, and other vegetables. Lecithin is unusual in that it is a naturally occurring amphoteric surfactant and emulsifying agent. Its amphoteric nature makes it substantive to hair. It is used mainly as a coemulsifier with another, more powerful, surfactant as the primary emulsifier. It has some antioxidant properties and greatly improves emulsion stability.

Class: Glyceryl Esters and Derivatives, Phosphorus Compounds

Function: Surfactants—Emulsifying Agent

Found in: Shampoos, Conditioners, Hairsprays, Setting Lotions, Hair Dyes, Hair Colorants, Permanent Waves, Hair Straighteners, Miscellaneous

Other Names: Soybean Phospholipid, Alpha-Phosphatidyl Choline

Linoleamide DEA (LIN-oh-lee-am-eyed DEA)

Definition: Linoleamide DEA is a mixture of diethanolamides of linoleic acid and has been unofficially called vitamin F. Although this nonionic surfactant is usually used in foaming preparations, it is also an excellent emollient and conditioner that improves wet combing and reduces static electricity.

Class: Alkanolamides

Function: Surfactants—Foam Booster, Conditioner

Found in: Shampoos, Conditioners, Hairsprays, Setting Lotions, Hair Dyes, Hair Colorants, Miscellaneous
Other Names: N-Linoleoyl Ethanolamine, Linoleic Acid Diethanolamide

Linoleic Acid (LIN-oh-ley-ik AS-ud)

Definition: Linoleic acid is an unsaturated fatty acid.
Class: Fatty Acids
Function: Conditioners—Moisturizer
Found in: Shampoos, Conditioners, Hair Dyes, Hair Colorants, Miscellaneous
Other Names: 9, 12-Octadecadienoic Acid

L

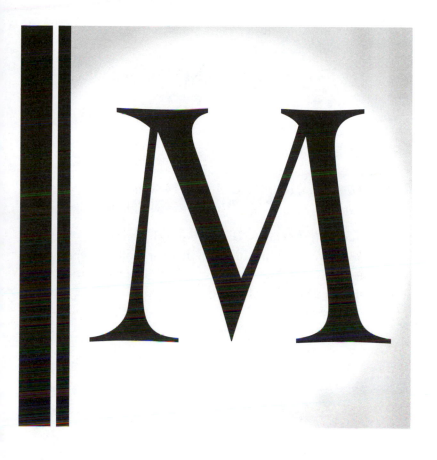

Magnesium Aluminum Silicate (mag-NEE-zee-um uh-LOO-min-um SIL-uh-kayt)

Definition: Magnesium aluminum silicate is a complex silicate refined from naturally occurring minerals. Clay minerals are known as smectrite clays that swell when water is added to form a gel. The addition of magnesium aluminum silicate causes a thicker, more stable emulsion.

Class: Inorganic Salts

Function: Thickener

Found in: Shampoos, Conditioners, Permanent Waves, Hair Straighteners, Hair Dyes, Hair Colorants, Miscellaneous

Other Names: Aluminum Magnesium Silicate, Silicic Acid Aluminum Magnesium Salt

Magnesium Lauryl Sulfate (mag-NEE-zee-um LOR-ul SUL-fayt)

Definition: Magnesium lauryl sulfate is the magnesium salt of lauryl sulfate.

Class: Alkyl Sulfates

Function: Surfactants—Cleansing Agent

Found in: Shampoos, Conditioners, Miscellaneous

Other Names: Magnesium Monododecyl Sulfate

Magnesium Sulfate (mag-NEE-zee-um SUL-fayt)

Definition: Magnesium sulfate is the inorganic salt commonly known as epsom salt. It is used in the pharmaceutical industry as a laxative. The natural sources of this ingredient are magnesium ores. It is used in hair care products to claim a natural mineral content and also because it acts as an astringent.

Class: Inorganic Salts

Function: Natural Mineral, Astringent

Found in: Shampoos, Conditioners, Miscellaneous

Other Names: Epsom Salt, Sulfuric Acid Magnesium Salt

Malic Acid (MAL-ik AS-ud)

Definition: Malic acid is a carboxylic acid used to adjust pH.

Class: Carboxylic Acids

Function: pH Adjuster

Found in: Shampoos, Conditioners, Miscellaneous

Other Names: Deoxytetraric Acid, Hydroxybutanedioic Acid, Hydroxysuccinnic Acid

MEA-Lauryl Sulfate (MEA-LOR-ul SUL-fayt)

Definition: MEA-lauryl sulfate is the monoethanolamine salt of sulfated lauryl alcohol.

Class: Alkyl Sulfates

Function: Surfactants—Cleansing Agent

Found in: Shampoos, Conditioners, Miscellaneous

Other Names: MEA-Dodecyl Sulfate, Monoethanolamine Lauryl Sulfate

Menthol (MEN-thawl)

Definition: Menthol is a diterpene that is found in oil of peppermint and other natural oils, and can be synthesized by the hydrogenation of thymol. It produces a cooling effect on the skin, but can be irritating to skin and eyes, especially at high concentrations.

Class: Alcohols

Function: Fragrance

Found in: Shampoos, Conditioners, Hair Straighteners, Miscellaneous

Other Names: Cyclohexanol, Racemic Menthol

Mercaptopropionic Acid (mer-KAP-toh-pro-pee-ohn-ik AS-ud)

Definition: Mercaptopropionic acid is a thio compound (mercaptan) used as a hair waving and straightening agent.

Class: Thio Compounds, Carboxylic Acids

Function: Hair Waving and Straightening — Reducing Agent

Found in: Permanent Waves, Hair Straighteners

Other Names: 2-Mercaptoethanecarboxylic Acid, Thiolatic Acid

Methacryloyl Ethyl Betaine/Acrylates Copolymer (METH-uh-kril-oil ETH-ul BEE-tayn/uh-KRIL-ayts koh-PAHL-uh-mur)

Definition: Methacryloyl ethyl betaine/acrylates copolymer is a polymer of methylacryloyl ethyl betaine and methacrylic acid or its simple esters.

Class: Synthetic Polymers

Function: Hair Fixatives

Found in: Hairsprays, Aerosol Hairsprays, Setting Lotions

Other Names: Methacryloyl Ethyl Betaine/Methacrylates Copolymer

Methenamine (METH-en-am-een)

Definition: Methenamine is an organic amine used as a preservative.

Class: Amines

Function: Preservative

Found in: Shampoos, Conditioners, Miscellaneous

Other Names: Aminoform, Formamine, Hexamethylene Tetramine, Methenamide, Methenamin

Methicone (METH-uh-kown)

Definition: Methicone is a linear monomethyl polysiloxane. This class of ingredients is generally referred to as silicones.

Class: Siloxanes and Silanes

Function: Conditioners — Moisturizers

Found in: Conditioners, Hair Dyes, Hair Colorants, Miscellaneous

Other Names: Hydrogen Methyl Polysiloxane

Methylchloroisothiazolinone (METH-ul-klohr-oh-eye-soh-thi-uh-zoh-lyn-own)

Definition: Methylchloroisothiazolinone is a heterocyclic organic compound used as a preservative. This ingredient is a powerful, broad-spectrum antimicrobial and antifungal agent.

Class: Heterocyclic Compounds

Function: Preservative

Found in: Shampoos, Conditioners, Setting Lotions, Permanent Waves, Hair Straighteners, Hair Dyes, Hair Colorants, Miscellaneous

Other Names: Chloromethylisothiazolinone

Methyl Hydroxyethylcellulose (METH-ul hy-DRAHKS-ee-eth-ul-sel-yu-lohs)

Definition: Methyl hydroxyethylcellulose is the methyl ether of hydroxyethylcellulose formed by reacting methylcellulose with ethylene oxide.

Class: Gums, Hydrophilic Colloids and Derivatives
Function: Thickener, Emulsion Stabilizer
Found in: Shampoos, Conditioners, Miscellaneous
Other Names: Hydroxyethylcellulose, Methylcellulose

Methylisothiazolinone (METH-ul-eye-soh-thy-uh-zoh-lyn-own)

Definition: Methylisothiazolinone is the heterocyclic organic preservative that is usually used in a blend with other preservatives to produce methylchloroisothiazolinone.
Class: Heterocyclic Compounds
Function: Preservative
Found in: Shampoos, Conditioners, Setting Lotions, Hair Dyes, Hair Colorants, Permanent Waves, Hair Straighteners, Miscellaneous
Other Names: Methylchloroisothiazolinone

Methylparaben (meth-ul-PAYR-uh-ben)

Definition: Methylparaben is the ester of methyl alcohol and p-hydroxybenzoic acid. It is effective against molds, yeast, and bacteria, and is usually used in combination with propylparaben because of the additive and synergistic effects.
Class: Esters, Phenols
Function: Preservative
Found in: Shampoos, Conditioners, Hairsprays, Setting Lotions, Hair Dyes, Hair Colorants, Permanent Waves, Hair Straighteners, Miscellaneous
Other Names: p-Carbomryhoxyphenol, Methyl Parahydroxybenzoate

Mica (MY-kuh)

Definition: Mica is a general term for a large group of naturally occurring hydrous silicates of aluminum and potassium (muscovite mica). Micas can be colorless or almost any color including black. Mica is coated with titanium dioxide when used as a pearling agent to provide optical effects ranging from a soft luster to sparkle.

Class: Inorganics, Colorants

Function: Colorant, Pearling Agent (with Titanium Dioxide)

Found in: Shampoos, Conditioners, Permanent Waves, Hair Straighteners, Hair Dyes, Hair Colorants, Miscellaneous

Other Names: Golden Mica, Muscovite Mica, Pigment White 20, Sericite

Microcrystalline Wax (my-kroh-KRYS-tuh-lyn WAKS)

Definition: Microcrystalline Wax is derived from petroleum and characterized by its fine crystals, in contrast with the larger crystals of paraffin wax.

Class: Hydrocarbons, Waxes

Function: Thickener, Bulking Agent

Found in: Setting Lotions, Styling Aids

Other Names: Cera Microcristallina, Petroleum Wax, Microcrystaline

Milk (MILK)

Definition: Milk is the whole milk obtained from cows. It consists of milk solids, fats, protein, and lactose. Milk has been used in personal care products for thousands of years, often with honey. Although it is currently used as a conditioner, its major appeal is the association with mildness, health, purity, and its historic use. It is unlikely that milk or milk protein has any significant benefit.

Class: Biological Products

Function: Conditioner

Found in: Shampoos, Conditioners, Miscellaneous

Other Names: Cow's Milk

Mineral Oil (MIN-ur-ul Oyl)

Definition: Mineral oil is a complex liquid mixture of paraffinic hydrocarbons obtained from petroleum. It is a colorless, odorless, highly stable, oily liquid that is considered nontoxic and nonirritating.

Class: Hydrocarbons

Function: Conditioners—Moisturizer

Found in: Shampoos, Conditioners, Permanent Waves, Hair Straighteners, Hair Dyes, Hair Colorants, Miscellaneous

Other Names: Deobase, Heavy Mineral Oil, Light Mineral Oil, Liquid Paraffin, Liquid Petroleum, Paraffin Oil, Prolatum Oil

Mink Oil (MINK OYL)

Definition: Mink oil is a natural oil obtained form the subdermal fatty tissues of the mink and a by-product of the mink fur industry. Mink oil is composed primarily of triglycerides of oleic, palmitoleic, palmitic, and linoleic fatty acids. It is the only natural ester of animal origin, besides lanolin, that is currently used since the ban on whale products.

Class: Fats and Oils

Function: Conditioners—Moisturizer

Found in: Shampoos, Conditioners, Permanent Waves, Hair Straighteners, Hair Dyes, Hair Colorants, Miscellaneous

Other Names: Mustela Oil, Oil of Mink

Myristalkonium Chloride (meer-uh-stal-KOHN-ee-um KHLOR-eyed)

Definition: Myristalkonium chloride is a quaternary ammonium salt. It is a powerful batericide, particularly in combination with Quaternium-14. It is similar to benzalkonium chloride, and although it has some conditioning effect, that is not the main reason for its use.

Class: Quaternary Ammonium Compounds

Function: Preservative, Conditioners—Antistatic

Found in: Shampoos, Conditioners, Permanent Waves, Hair Straighteners, Hair Dyes, Hair Colorants, Miscellaneous

Other Names: Myristyl Dimethylbenzylammonium Chloride, Benzyldimethyltetradecylammonium Chloride, Miristalkonium Chloride

Myristyl Alcohol (MEER-uh-stil AL-kuh-hawl)

Definition: Myristyl alcohol is a fatty alcohol (C-14) that is used in hair care products for a wide variety of reasons.

Class: Fatty Alcohols

Function: Surfactants — Foam Booster, Thickener, Emulsion Stabilizer

Found in: Hair Dyes, Hair Colorants, Miscellaneous

Other Names: 1-Hydroxytetradecane, Tetradecanol, Tetradecyl Alcohol

Myristyl Myristate (MEER-uh-stil MEER-uh-stayt)

Definition: Myristyl myristate is the ester of myristyl alcohol and myristic acid.

Class: Esters

Function: Conditioners — Moisturizer

Found in: Shampoos, Conditioners, Miscellaneous

Other Names: Tetradecanoic Acid, Tetradecyl Ester, Tetradecyl Tetradecanoate

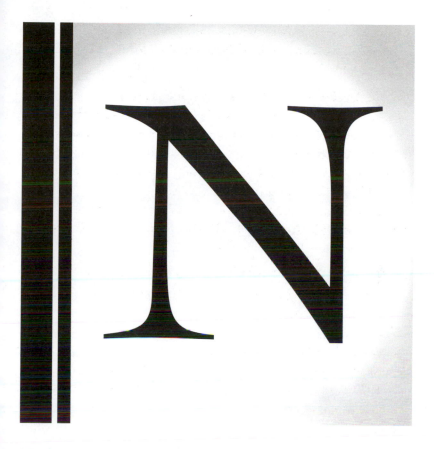

Niacinamide (NYE-uh-sin-am-eyed)

Definition: Niacinamide is a heterocyclic aromatic amide and is the amide form of the vitamin sometimes called niacin (nicotinic acid). Both the acid and amide forms are found in minute quantities in living cells, and their absence is associated with pellagra. It is obtained commercially by the oxidation of 3-cyanopyridine and the oxidation of nicotine.

The names niacin and niacinamide were coined because they were felt to be more acceptable to the public than nicotinic acid and nicotinamide. Although it is reported to stimulate hair growth, there is no evidence to this effect. It is usually added because of its sales appeal as a natural vitamin.

Class: Amides, Heterocyclic Compounds
Function: Conditioners—Miscellaneous
Found in: Shampoos, Conditioners, Miscellaneous
Other Names: Nicotininic Acid Amide, Vitamin B-3,
   3-Pyridinecarboxamide

Nitrophenol (NYE-troh-feh-nawl)

Definition: Nitrophenol is a substituted phenol used as a hair
   colorant. Numerous variations of this ingredient are used in
   haircoloring to produce a wide variety of different colors.
Class: Phenols
Function: Hair Colorant
Found in: Hair Dyes, Hair Colorants
Other Names: Mononitrophenol

4-Nitro-o-Phenylenediamine (NYE-troh-oh-FEN-ul-een-deye-am-een)

Definition: 4-nitro-o-phenylenediamine is a substituted aromatic amine used as a hair colorant. Numerous variations
   of this ingredient are used in haircoloring to produce a
   wide variety of different colors.
Class: Amines
Function: Hair Colorant
Found in: Hair Dyes, Hair Colorants
Other Names: 2-Amino-4-Nitroaniline, 1,2-Benzenediamine
   4-Nitro

Nonoxynol-10 (no-NAHKS-ee-nawl)

Definition: Nonoxynol-10 is an ethoxylated alkyl phenol prepared by ethoxylation of a mixture of monoalkyl phenols
   and an ethoxylation value of 10. Varying degrees of
   ethoxylation produce similar ingredients with slightly different characteristics. This is an inexpensive nonionic surfactant that is frequently used in dishwashing liquids as a
   foaming and cleansing agent.
Class: Alkoxylated Alcohols

Function: Surfactants — Emulsifying Agent

Found in: Shampoos, Conditioners, Hairsprays, Setting Lotions, Hair Dyes, Hair Colorants, Permanent Waves, Hair Straighteners, Miscellaneous

Other Names: PEG-10 Nonyl Phenyl Ether, Polyethylene Glycol 500 Nonyl Phenyl Ether, Polyoxyethylene (10) Nonylphenol Ether, Decaethylene Glycol Nonylohenyl Ether

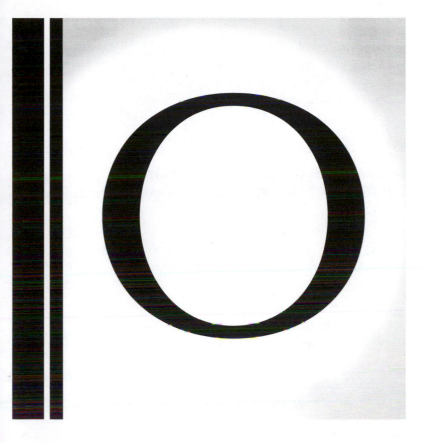

Octoxynol-9 (AHKT-ahks-ee-nawl)

Definition: Octoxynol-9 is an ethoxylated alkyl phenol with an ethoxylation value of 9. It is similar to nonoxynol-10, but less biodegradable. It is an inexpensive nonionic surfactant used primarily as an emulsifying agent.

Class: Alkoxylated Alcohols

Function: Surfactants—Emulsifying Agent

Found in: Shampoos, Conditioners, Hairsprays, Setting Lotions, Hair Dyes, Hair Colorants, Permanent Waves, Hair Straighteners, Miscellaneous

Other Names: PEG-9 Octyl Phenyl Ether, Polyethylene Glycol 450 Octyl Phenyl Ether

Octyldodecanol (ahk-tul-doh-DEK-un-awl)

Definition: Octyldodecanol is an aliphatic fatty alcohol.

Class: Alcohols

Function: Conditioners—Moisturizer

Found in: Shampoos, Conditioners, Hairsprays, Setting Lotions, Hair Dyes, Hair Colorants, Miscellaneous

Other Names: 2-Octyldodecyl Alcoho

Oleamide DEA (OH-lee-am-eyed DEA)

Definition: Oleamide DEA is a mixture of ethanolamides of oleic acid and is often produced from olive oil. Oleamide DEA has many of the properties of cocamide DEA, but provides superior conditioning. This ingredient is also a good thickener, foam booster, and foam stabilizer.

Class: Alkanolamides

Function: Surfactants—Foam Booster, Stabilizer, Thickener

Found in: Shampoos, Conditioners, Hair Dyes, Hair Colorants, Miscellaneous

Other Names: Diethanolamine Oleic Acid Amide, Oleic Diethanolamide, Oleylamide DEA

Oleic Acid (oh-LEY-ik AS-ud)

Definition: Oleic acid is an unsaturated fatty acid that is anionic when neutralized and is often produced from olive oil, which contains about 80 percent oleic acid. It is more substantive to the hair than stearic acid because it is unsaturated.

Class: Fatty Acids

Function: Thickener, Conditioners—Moisturizer, Surfactants—Foam Booster

Found in: Shampoos, Conditioners, Permanent Waves, Hair Straighteners, Hair Dyes, Hair Colorants, Miscellaneous

Other Names: 9-Octadecenoic Acid

Oleth-10 (OH-leth-10)

Definition: Oleth-10 is a polyethylene glycol ether of oleyl alcohol with an ethoxylation value of 10. This is a nonionic emulsifying agent. Oleyl alcohol ethoxylates are mild emollients that are slightly substantive to hair and skin. Varying degrees of ethoxylation produce similar ingredients with slightly varied characteristics.

Class: Alkoxylated Alcohols

Function: Surfactants—Emulsifying Agent, Conditioner

Found in: Shampoos, Conditioners, Hair Dyes, Hair Colorants, Miscellaneous

Other Names: Decaethylene Glycol Monooleyl Ether, PEG-10 Oleyl Ether, Polyoxyethylene (10) Oleyl Ether

Oleyl Alcohol (OH-ley-ul AL-kuh-hawl)

Definition: Oleyl alcohol is an unsaturated fatty alcohol obtained from oleic acid or methyl oleate from tallow, olive oil, canola oil, palm oil, and tall oil. It is similar to cetyl alcohol, but is slightly more substantive and a more effective conditioner because it is unsaturated.

Class: Fatty Alcohols

Function: Conditioners—Moisturizer, Emulsifying Agent

Found in: Shampoos, Conditioners, Hairsprays, Setting Lotions, Hair Dyes, Hair Colorants, Permanent Waves, Hair Straighteners, Miscellaneous

Other Names: cis-9-Octadecenyl Alcohol, Oleic Alcohol

Ozokerite (oh-zoh-KER-eyt)

Definition: Ozokerite is a naturally occurring mineral hydrocarbon wax derived from mineral or petroleum sources.

Class: Waxes

Function: Thickener, Emulsion Stabilizer

Found in: Hair Dyes, Hair Colorants, Miscellaneous

Other Names: Ozocerite Wax

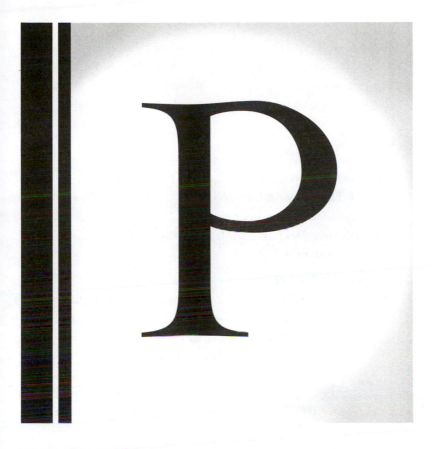

PABA (PAH-buh)

Definition: PABA (para-amino benzoic acid) is an aromatic acid that is part of the vitamin B complex. Although it is not regarded as a vitamin, it is part of the folic acid molecule, which is a vitamin. It has been reported to cause sensitization with repeated exposure, and allergic reactions in predisposed individuals. It is used as a UV-B sunscreen.

Class: Amines, Amino Acids

Function: Sunscreen

Found in: Shampoos, Conditioners, Hairsprays, Setting Lotions

Other Names: Para-Amino Benzoic Acid, Aminobenzoic Acid

Panthenol (PAN-thuh-nawl)

Definition: Panthenol is the DL form of pantothenyl alcohol and dexpanthenol that are the vitamin forms. Panthenol is a pro-vitamin, or precursor, of pantothenic acid, which is also known as vitamin B-5. Panthenol adds pliability and luster to hair.

Class: Alcohols, Amides

Function: Conditioner

Found in: Shampoos, Conditioners, Hairsprays, Setting Lotions, Hair Dyes, Hair Colorants, Permanent Waves, Hair Straighteners, Miscellaneous

Other Names: Dexpanthenol, Pantothenol, Pantothenyl Alcohol, Provitamin B-5

Paraffin (PAYR-uh-fin)

Definition: Paraffin is a complex mixture of solid, mainly straight chain hydrocarbons derived from petroleum. Paraffin's main function is to alter the physical characteristics of the product and produce a thicker product than possible with oils alone. Although paraffin wax is a mineral and natural material, it does not have the right image as a natural ingredient since it is derived from petroleum

Class: Hydrocarbons, Waxes

Function: Thickener, Conditioners — Moisturizer

Found in: Conditioners, Styling Lotions, Hair Dyes, Hair Colorants, Miscellaneous

Other Names: Petroleum Wax, Crystalline Waxes, Paraffin Oil, Liquid Paraffin

Pectin (PEK-tin)

Definition: Pectin is the purified carbohydrate extracted from the inner portion of the rind of citrus fruits or from apples. It consists chiefly of partially methoxylated polygalacturonic acids.

Class: Gums, Hydrophilic Compounds

Function: Thickener

Found in: Shampoos, Conditioners, Hairsprays, Setting Lotions, Permanent Waves, Hair Straighteners, Miscellaneous

Other Names: Citrus Pectin

PEG-8 (PEG-8)

Definition: PEG-8 is the polymer of ethylene oxide with an average value of 8.

Class: Alkoxylated Alcohols, Polymeric Ethers

Function: Conditioners—Humectant

Found in: Shampoos, Conditioners, Miscellaneous

Other Names: Polyethylene Glycol, Polyoxyethylene, Octaethylene Glycol

PEG-40 Castor Oil (PEG-40 KAS-tohr OYL)

Definition: PEG-40 castor oil is a polyethylene glycol derivative of *Ricinus communis* (castor oil) with an ethoxylation value of 40. This natural oil contains a very high percentage of glyceryl triricinoleate. PEG-40 castor oil is a very mild nonionic emulsifier with good moisturizing and emollient properties.

Class: Alkoxylated Alcohols, Glyceryl Esters and Derivatives

Function: Surfactants—Emulsifying Agent, Conditioners—Moisturizer

Found in: Permanent Waves, Straighteners, Conditioners, Miscellaneous

Other Names: Polyethylene Glycol 2000 Castor Oil, Polyoxyethylene (40) Castor Oil

PEG-150 Dilaurate (PEG-150 dy-LOR-ayt)

Definition: PEG-150 dilaurate is a polyethylene glycol diester of lauric acid with an ethoxylation value of 150. This emulsifier has a thickening effect and also acts as a solubilizer for some oils. PEG esters are typically very mild and can reduce the irritation of other ingredients.

Class: Alkoxylated Carboxylic Acids

Function: Surfactants — Emulsifier, Conditioners —
Moisturizer
Found in: Conditioners, Miscellaneous
Other Names: Polyethylene Glycol 6000 Dilaurate, Poly-
oxyethylene (150) Dilaurate

PEG-4 Distearate (PEG-4-dy-STEER-ayt)
Definition: PEG-4 distearate is the polyethylene glycol
diester of stearic acid with an ethoxylation value of 4. This
nonionic emulsifier has conditioning and thickening
properties.
Class: Alkoxylated Carboxylic Acids
Function: Surfactants — Emulsifying Agent, Thickener
Found in: Conditioners, Miscellaneous
Other Names: Polyethylene Glycol 200 Distearate, Poly-
oxyethylene (4) Distearate

PEG-7 Glyceryl Cocoate (PEG-7-GLIS-ur-il KOH-koh-ayt)
Definition: PEG-7 glyceryl cocoate is the polyethylene glycol
ether of glyceryl cocoate derived from coconut oil with an
ethoxylation value of 7. This extremely mild, nonionic
emulsifier is prepared by ethoxylation of glyceryl monococoate. It is used as a conditioner and solubilizer for essential oils.
Class: Alkoxylated Alcohols, Glyceryl Esters and Derivatives
Function: Conditioners — Moisturizer, Surfactants —
Emulsifier
Found in: Shampoos, Conditioners, Hair Dyes, Hair Colorants, Miscellaneous
Other Names: Polyethylene Glycol (7) Glyceryl Monococoate, Polyoxyethylene (7) Glyceryl Monococoate

PEG-40 Hydrogenated Castor Oil (PEG-40 HY-druh-jen-ayt-ud KAS-tohr OYL)
Definition: PEG-40 hydrogenated castor oil is a polyethylene
glycol derivative of hydrogenated castor oil with an

ethoxylation value of 40. This mild, nonionic emulsifier is similar to PEG-40 castor oil and is prepared by hydrogenation of castor oil to produce glyceryl trihydroxystearate prior to ethoxylation.

Class: Alkoxylated Alcohols, Glyceryl Esters and Derivatives

Function: Surfactants — Emulsifier, Conditioners — Moisturizer

Found in: Shampoos, Conditioners, Hairsprays, Setting Lotions, Miscellaneous

Other Names: Polyethylene Glycol 2000 Hydrogenated Castor Oil, Polyoxyethylene (40) Hydrogenated Castor Oil

PEG-75 Lanolin (PEG-75 LAN-ul-un)

Definition: PEG-75 lanolin is a polyethylene glycol derivative of Lanolin with an ethoxylation value of 75. This nonionic emulsifier has some of the conditioning properties of lanolin and also functions as an anti-irritant.

Class: Alkoxylated Alcohols, Lanolin and Lanolin Derivatives

Function: Surfactants — Emulsifier, Conditioners — Moisturizer

Found in: Shampoos, Conditioners, Hair Dyes, Hair Colorants, Permanent Waves, Hair Straighteners, Miscellaneous

Other Names: Polyethylene Glycol 4000 Lanolin, Polyoxyethylene (75) Lanolin

PEG-44 Sorbitan Laurate (PEG-44 SOR-buh-tan LOR-ayt)

Definition: PEG-44 sorbitan laurate is an ethoxylated sorbitan ester of lauric acid with an ethoxylation value of 40. This nonionic surfactant is used as a mild foaming and cleansing agent, and anti-irritant.

Class: Sorbitan Derivatives

Function: Surfactants — Cleansing Agent, Foam Booster

Found in: Shampoos, Conditioners, Hairsprays, Setting Lotions, Hair Dyes, Hair Colorants, Permanent Waves, Hair Straighteners, Miscellaneous

Other Names: Polyethylene Glycol (44) Sorbitan Monolaurate, Polyoxyethylene (75) Sorbitan Monolaurate

PEG-5 Soy Sterol (PEG-5- SOY STER-awl)

Definition: PEG-5 soy sterol is a polyethylene glycol derivative of the phytosterols found in glycine soja (soybean oil) with an ethoxylation value of 5. Although ethoxylated soy sterols are substantive to hair, the substantivity decreases with higher degrees of ethoxylation.

Class: Alkoxylated Alcohols, Sterols

Function: Surfactants—Emulsifying Agent, Conditioners— Moisturizer

Found in: Conditioners, Miscellaneous

Other Names: PEG-5 Soya Sterol, Polyethylene Glycol (5) Soy Sterol, Polyoxyethylene (5) Soy Sterol

PEG-100 Stearate (PEG-100 STEER-ayt)

Definition: PEG-100 stearate is the polyethylene glycol ester of stearic acid with an ethoxylation value of 100. This non-ionic surfactant is used as an emulsifier, conditioner, and thickener. PEG-esters are very mild and may reduce the irritation of other ingredients.

Class: Alkoxylated Carboxylic Acids

Function: Surfactants—Emulsifier, Conditioners— Moisturizer, Thickener

Found in: Conditioner, Miscellaneous

Other Names: Polyethylene Glycol 100 Monostearate, Polyoxyethylene (100) Monostearate

Pentasodium Pentetate (pent-uh-SOH-dee-um PENT-uh-tayt)

Definition: Pentasodium pentetate is the pentasodium salt of diethylenetriaminepentaacetic acid.

Class: Amines, Organic Salts

Function: Chelating Agent

Found in: Setting Lotions, Permanent Waves, Hair Straighteners, Hair Dyes, Hair Colorants, Miscellaneous

Other Names: Pentasodium Diethylenetriaminepentaacetate

Petrolatum (peh-TROH-lat-um)

Definition: Petrolatum is a complex, semisolid mixture of wax-like and high molecular weight hydrocarbons obtained from petroleum. A number of grades are available that differ by color, melting point, and consistency. Petrolatum is used in conditioners because it forms an occlusive, water-impenetrable, film on skin and hair.

Class: Hydrocarbons

Function: Conditioners—Moisturizer, Thickener

Found in: Shampoos, Conditioners, Setting Lotions, Permanent Waves, Hair Straighteners, Hair Dyes, Hair Colorants, Miscellaneous

Other Names: Mineral Jelly, Petrolatum Amber, Petrolatum White, Petrolatum Jelly, White Petrolatum, Yellow Petrolatum

Phenoxyethanol (fen-AHKS-ee-eth-an-awl)

Definition: Phenoxyethanol is an aromatic ether alcohol used as a preservative, solvent, and fragrance. It is usually mixed with parabens for use as a broad-spectrum preservative. It is a powerful solvent with a rose-like odor and is used as a perfume fixative.

Class: Alcohols, Ethers

Function: Preservative, Solvent, Fragrance

Found in: Shampoos, Conditioners, Hairsprays, Setting Lotions, Permanent Waves, Hair Straighteners, Hair Dyes, Hair Colorants, Miscellaneous

Other Names: Ethylene Glycol Monophenyl Ether, 2-Phenoxyethanol, Phenoxytol

p-Phenylenediamine (PAIR-uh FEN-ul-een-dy-am-een)

Definition: p-phenylenediamine is an aromatic amine used as a haircolorant and is exempt from regulation as a hair dye.

Class: Amines, Hair Colorants

Function: Hair Colorant

Found in: Hair Dyes, Hair Colorants
Other Names: p-aminoaniline, 1,4-Benzenediamine

Phenyl Trimethicone (FEN-ul try-METH-uh-kohn)

Definition: Phenyl trimethicone is a siloxane polymer used as a conditioner and antifoaming agent.
Class: Siloxanes and Silanes
Function: Conditioners—Moisturizer
Found in: Conditioners, Hairsprays, Setting Lotions, Hair Dyes, Hair Colorants, Miscellaneous
Other Names: None Available

Phosphoric Acid (FAHS-fohr-ik AS-ud)

Definition: Phosphoric acid is an inorganic acid obtained industrially from phosphate rock deposits where it occurs as tricalcium phosphate. It is used as a flavor in soft drinks and is generally recognized as safe. It is used in hair care products to adjust pH.
Class: Inorganic Acids
Function: pH Adjuster
Found in: Shampoos, Conditioners, Hairsprays, Setting Lotions, Permanent Waves, Hair Straighteners, Hair Dyes, Hair Colorants, Miscellaneous
Other Names: Hydrogen Phosphate, Orthophosphoric Acid

Phytantriol (Fy-tan-TREE-awl)

Definition: Phytantriol is an aliphatic alcohol. It is a diterpene with a repeating isoprene pattern and is related to the tetramethyl monounsaturated C20 primary alcohol phytol.
Class: Polyols
Function: Conditioners—Moisturizer
Found in: Shampoos, Conditioners, Hairsprays, Setting Lotions, Miscellaneous
Other Names: Tetramethyl Trihydroxyhexadecane

Pigment Blue 15 (PIG-mint BLOO 15)

Definition: Pigment blue 15 is a phthalocyanine (copper complex) color.

Class: Hair Colorant

Function: Hair Colorant

Found in: Hair Dyes, Hair Colorants

Other Names: Blue No. 404, Copper Phthalocyanine, Heliogen Blue B

Poloxamer 101 (PAHL-ahks-uh-mur 101)

Definition: Poloxamer 101 is a polyoxyethylene, polyoxypropylene block polymer formed by condensing 16 moles of propylene oxide followed by four moles of ethylene oxide. It is nontoxic, but is a mild sensitizer in individuals predisposed to allergies.

Class: Polymeric Ethers

Function: Surfactants—Emulsifying Agent, Thickener

Found in: Shampoos, Conditioners, Miscellaneous

Other Names: None Available

Polyacrylamide (pahl-ee-uh-KRIL-am-eyed)

Definition: Polyacrylamide is a synthetic polymer of acrylamide monomers, or a copolymer of acrylamide and sodium acrylate. It is used as an emulsion stabilizer, thickener, and detoxifying agent.

Class: Amides, Synthetic Polymers

Function: Thickener

Found in: Conditioners, Hair Dyes, Hair Colorants, Miscellaneous

Other Names: Acrylamide Homopolymer, 2-Propenamide Homopolymer

Polyquaternium-10 (pahl-ee-KWAT-ur-nee-um 10)

Definition: Polyquaternium-10 is a polymeric quaternary ammonium salt of hydroxyethylcellulose reacted with a trimethyl ammonium substituted epoxide. This cationic polymer is a film-forming, water-soluble resin that is substantive to hair and improves wet-combing, curl retention, and flyaway hair.

Class: Quaternary Ammonium Compounds, Synthetic Polymers

Function: Conditioners—Antistatic

Found in: Shampoos, Conditioners, Hairsprays, Setting Lotions, Permanent Waves, Hair Straighteners, Hair Dyes, Hair Colorants, Miscellaneous

Other Names: Quaternium-19

Polysorbate 20 (pahl-ee-SOR-bayt 20)

Definition: Polysorbate 20 is a mixture of laurate esters of sorbitol and sorbitol anhydrides, condensed with 20 moles of ethylene oxide. This mild foaming and cleansing agent also reduces the irritation of other ingredients.

Class: Sorbitan Derivatives

Function: Surfactants—Emulsifying Agent

Found in: Shampoos, Conditioners, Hairsprays, Setting Lotions, Permanent Waves, Hair Straighteners, Hair Dyes, Hair Colorants, Miscellaneous

Other Names: Polyoxyethylene Sorbitan Monolaurate, Sorbimacrogol Laurate

Potassium Chloride (poh-TAS-ee-um KLOHR-eyed)

Definition: Potassium chloride is an inorganic salt used in small quantities to make minor adjustments in a product's viscosity. It is considered harmless.

Class: Inorganic Salts

Function: Thickener

Found in: Shampoos, Conditioners, Miscellaneous

Other Names: None Available

Potassium Cocoate (poh-TAS-ee-um koh-KOH-ayt)

Definition: Potassium cocoate is the potassium salt of coconut fatty acid. It is a foaming and cleansing agent that is usually prepared by saponifying coconut oil with potassium hydroxide. Although coconut fatty acid soaps are good foaming agents, they are poor cleansers.

Class: Soaps
Function: Surfactants—Foam Booster, Cleansing Agent
Found in: Shampoos, Conditioners, Miscellaneous
Other Names: None Available

Potassium Hydroxide (poh-TAS-ee-um hy-DRAHKS-eyed)

Definition: Potassium hydroxide is an inorganic alkali that is used to neutralize acids and increase the pH of a product.
Class: Inorganic Alkalis
Function: pH Adjuster
Found in: Shampoos, Aerosol Hairsprays, Miscellaneous
Other Names: Caustic Potash

Potassium Metabisulfite (poh-TAS-ee-um met-uh-by-SUL-fyt)

Definition: Potassium metabisulfite is an inorganic salt and a reducing agent that is used in hair waving and straightening.
Class: Inorganic Salts
Function: Hair Waving and Straightening—Reducing Agent
Found in: Permanent Waves, Hair Straighteners
Other Names: Dipotassium Disulfite, Dipotassium Pyrosulfate, Potassium Pyrosulfite

Potassium Oleate (poh-TAS-ee-um OH-lee-ayt)

Definition: Potassium oleate is the potassium salt of oleic acid. This soap is used as an emulsifying agent.
Class: Soaps
Function: Surfactants—Emulsifying Agent
Found in: Permanent Waves, Hair Dyes, Hair Colorants
Other Names: Potassium 9-Octadecenoate

Potassium Persulfate (poh-TAS-ee-um pur-SUL-fayt)

Definition: Potassium persulfate is an inorganic salt used in powdered, off-the-scalp hair lighteners and hair bleaches. Although it significantly increases lightening ability, it is

P

usually only used in off-the-scalp products because it also causes scalp irritation.

Class: Inorganic Salts

Function: Oxidizer

Found in: Powdered Hair Lighteners and Bleaches

Other Names: Peroxydisulfuric Acid, Dipotassium Salt

Potassium Sorbate (poh-TAS-ee-um SOR-bayt)

Definition: Potassium sorbate is an organic salt used as a fungicide and antioxidant. It is also used as a preservative in foods and is generally considered safe. It is practically nontoxic and nonirritating.

Class: Organic Salts

Function: Preservative

Found in: Shampoos, Conditioners, Hair Dyes, Hair Colorants, Miscellaneous

Other Names: 2,4-Hexadienoic Acid, Potassium Salt

Potassium Sulfite (poh-TAS-ee-um SUL-fyt)

Definition: Potassium sulfite is an inorganic salt used as a reducing agent and antioxidant.

Class: Inorganic Salts

Function: Hair Waving and Straightening—Reducing Agents, Antioxidant

Found in: Permanent Waves, Hair Straighteners

Other Names: Sulfurous Acid, Potassium Salt

Potassium Thioglycolate (poh-TAS-ee-um thy-oh-GLY-kuh-layt)

Definition: Potassium thioglycolate is an organic salt and thio compound. It is used as a reducing agent in hair waving and straightening products. It may also be used, at a higher pH, as a depilating agent.

Class: Organic Salts, Thio Compounds

Function: Hair Waving and Straightening—Reducing Agents

Found in: Permanent Waves, Hair Straighteners

Other Names: Potassium Mercaptoacetate

PPG-9

Definition: PPG-9 is a polymer of propylene oxide. It is relatively nontoxic and nonirritating to skin. Polypropylene oxide compounds of high molecular weight reduce the irritation of other materials.

Class: Alkoxylated Alcohols, Polymeric Ethers

Function: Conditioners — Moisturizer

Found in: Shampoos, Miscellaneous

Other Names: Polyoxypropylene (9), Polypropylene Glycol (9)

PPG-2-Buteth-3 (PPG-2-BYOOT-eth-3)

Definition: PPG-2-buteth-3 is a polyoxypropylene, polyoxyethylene ether of butyl alcohol. It is used in a number of products as a water soluble lubricant and conditioner.

Class: Alkoxylated Alcohols

Function: Conditioners — Moisturizer

Found in: Shampoos, Conditioners, Miscellaneous

Other Names: Polyoxypropylene (2) Polyoxyethylene (3) monobutyl Ether

P

PPG-2 Lanolin Alcohol Ether (PPG-2 LAN-ul-un AL-kuh-hawl EETH-ur)

Definition: PPG-2 lanolin alcohol ether is the polypropylene glycol ether of lanolin alcohol. This propoxylated lanolin alcohol derivative is a nonionic surfactant that is used as an emollient, conditioner, and a coemulsifier.

Class: Alkoxylated Alcohols, Lanolin Derivatives

Function: Conditioners — Moisturizer

Found in: Shampoos, Conditioners, Miscellaneous

Other Names: Polyoxypropylene (2) Lanolin Ether, PPG-2 Lanolin Ether

PPG-10 Methyl Glucose Ether (PPG-10 METH-ul GLU-kohs EETH-ur)

Definition: PPG-10 methyl glucose ether is the polypropylene glycol ether of methyl glucose.

Class: Alkoxylated Alcohols, Carbohydrates

Function: Conditioners—Moisturizer

Found in: Hairsprays, Aerosol Hairsprays, Miscellaneous

Other Names: Polyoxypropylene (10) Methyl Glucose Ether

PPG-26 Oleate (PPG-26 OH-lee-ayt)

Definition: PPG-26 oleate is the polypropylene glycol ester of oleic acid.

Class: Alkoxylated Carboxylic Acids

Function: Conditioners—Moisturizer

Found in: Hairsprays, Aerosol Hairsprays, Miscellaneous

Other Names: Polyoxypropylene (26) Monooleate

Proline (PROH-leen)

Definition: Proline is a naturally occurring amino acid that is considered harmless.

Class: Amino Acids, Heterocyclic Compounds

Function: Conditioners—Moisturizer

Found in: Hair Conditioners, Permanent Waves

Other Names: L-Proline, 2-Pyrrolidine Carboxylic Acid

Propane (PROH-payn)

Definition: Propane is a colorless, explosive gas. This hydrocarbon is used as a propellant in aerosol hairsprays. It is usually used in combination with butane and isobutane. It does not deplete ozone in the atmosphere and is chemically inert, but it is flammable. It is generally recognized as safe and is also used as a propellant and aerating agent in food products.

Class: Hydrocarbons

Function: Propellant

Found in: Aerosols and Aerosol Hairsprays
Other Names: Dimethyl Methane

Propylene Glycol (PROH-pil-een GLY-kawl)

Definition: Propylene glycol is an aliphatic alcohol. It is completely water-soluble and used to moisturize and soften hair. It is also used as a solvent for some colors and other water-insoluble ingredients, and has some antimicrobial properties. Propylene glycol is considered harmless and is used in foods and hair care products to prevent them from drying out.

Class: Alcohols

Function: Conditioners — Humectant

Found in: Shampoos, Conditioners, Hairsprays, Setting Lotions, Hair Dyes, Hair Colorants, Miscellaneous

Other Names: 1,2-Propylene Glycol, Methyl Glycol, 1,2-Propanediol

Propylene Glycol Dicaprylate/Dicaprate (PROH-pil-een GLY-kawl dy-KAP-rill-ayt dy-KAP-rayt)

Definition: Propylene glycol dicaprylate/dicaprate is a mixture of the propylene glycol diesters of caprylic and capric acids.

Class: Esters

Function: Conditioners — Moisturizer

Found in: Shampoos, Conditioners, Miscellaneous

Other Names: Decanoic Acid, Mixed Diesters with Octanoic Acid and Propylene Glycol

Propylene Glycol Stearate (PROH-pil-een GLY-kawl STEER-ayt)

Definition: Propylene glycol stearate is the ester of propylene glycol and stearic acid. It is a waxy solid, which is not soluble in water. It is a weak nonionic surfactant that is used as a conditioner, hair softener, and coemulsifier.

Class: Esters

Function: Conditioners—Moisturizer, Surfactants—
Emulsifier

Found in: Shampoos, Conditioners, Miscellaneous

Other Names: Propylene Glycol Monostearate

Propylparaben (proh-pil-PAYR-a-ben)

Definition: Propylparaben is the ester of n-propyl alcohol and
p-hydroxybenzoic acid. It is a safe, odorless, colorless antimicrobial, which is often used in a blend with methylparaben. It is effective against molds, yeast, and bacteria,
and is nonirritating to skin and eyes.

Class: Esters, Phenols

Function: Preservative

Found in: Shampoos, Conditioners, Hairsprays, Setting Lotions, Hair Dyes, Hair Colorants, Miscellaneous

Other Names: Propyl p-Hydroxybenzoate, 4-Hydroxyben-
zoic Acid, Propyl Ester

PVP

Definition: PVP is a linear polymer that consists of 1-vinyl-2-
pyrrolidone monomers.

Class: Synthetic Polymers

Function: Hair Fixative

Found in: Shampoos, Conditioners, Hairsprays, Aerosol
Hairsprays, Setting Lotions

Other Names: Polyvinylpyrrolidone, Povidone

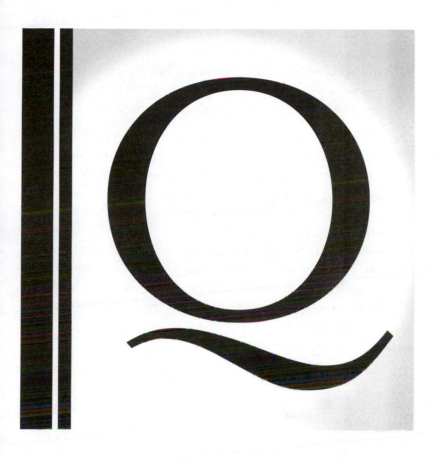

Quaternium-15 (kwah-TAYR-nee-um 15)

Definition: Quaternium-15 is a quaternary ammonium salt
that is highly active and used specifically as a broad-
spectrum antimicrobial. Although many other
quaternaries are used as conditioners, quaternium
15 has no fat chain and no conditioning properties.
It is slightly toxic and may be irritating to the eyes,
but is not irritating to skin. It is often used in
combination with parabens for complete antimicrobial
protection.

Class: Quaternary Ammonium Compounds

Function: Preservative

Found in: Shampoos, Conditioners, Hairsprays, Setting Lotions, Hair Dyes, Hair Colorants, Permanent Waves, Hair Straighteners, Miscellaneous

Other Names: Methenamine 3-Chloroallychloride

Quaternium 18 (kwah-TAYR-nee-um)

Definition: Quaternium 18 is a quaternary ammonium salt. Quaternary ammonium compounds are positively charged (cationic) and are substantive to the hair because they are attracted to the negative charges on hair. Many quaternary ammonium compounds are used as conditioning agents, especially in leave-in, antistatic conditioners. Quaternaries tend to be an irritant, and some are sensitizers. Quaternium 18 is a mild, but strongly cationic, hair conditioning agent, which helps reduce the static electricity that causes flyaway hair.

Class: Quaternary Ammonium Compounds

Function: Conditioners—Antistatic

Found in: Shampoos, Conditioners, Hairsprays, Setting Lotions, Hair Dyes, Hair Colorants, Permanent Waves, Hair Straighteners, Miscellaneous

Other Names: Dimethyl Di (Hydrogentated Tallow) Ammonium Chloride

Q

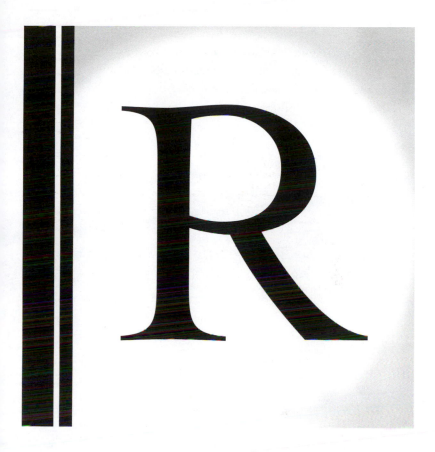

RED 4 (RED 4)

Definition: RED 4 is a monoazo color certified by the FDA for use in hair care products.

Class: Certified Color Additives

Function: Colorant

Found in: Shampoos, Conditioners, Setting Lotions, Hair Straighteners

Other Names: FD&C Red No. 4

Resorcinol (ree-SOHR-sin-awl)

Definition: Resorcinol is a phenol that is used in hair care products for a variety of different reasons. It is often used in hair colorants as a hair dye. Resorcinol may also be used as an external analgesic and is used as the active ingredient (drug) in antiacne products.

Class: Phenols

Function: Hair Colorant

Found in: Hair Dyes, Hair Colorants

Other Names: 1,3-Benzenediol, m-Dihydroxybenzene, m-Hydroquinone

Retinol (RET-in-awl)

Definition: Retinol is a component of vitamin A. The absence of this fat-soluble vitamin is associated with poor eyesight, and dry, chapped skin. Retinol is not very stable so it is usually used in hair care products in the more stable form of its palmitate ester (*see* Retinyl Palmitate).

Class: Alcohol

Function: Conditioners—Moisturizer

Found in: Shampoos, Conditioners, Miscellaneous

Other Names: Vitamin A

Retinyl Palmitate (RET-in-il PAHL-mu-tayt)

Definition: Retinyl palmitate is the ester of retinol and palmitic acid. This ester is more stable to oxidation than retinol and also has vitamin activity. It is often used in combination with ergocalciferol.

Class: Esters

Function: Conditioners—Moisturizer

Found in: Shampoos, Conditioners, Hairsprays, Setting Lotions, Hair Dyes, Hair Colorants, Miscellaneous

Other Names: Vitamin A Palmitate, Retinol Palmitate

R

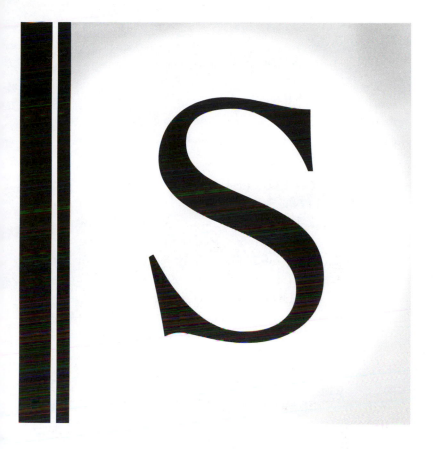

Salicylic Acid (sal-uh-SIL-ik AS-ud)

Definition: Salicylic acid is an aromatic acid that occurs in the form of esters in various plants such as methyl salicylate in oil of wintergreen. Salicylic acid may be used as an active ingredient (drug) in over-the-counter antidandruff shampoos. Although it is slightly toxic, it is used in foods as a preservative because of its antifungal properties.

Class: Carboxylic Acids, Phenols

Function: Antidandruff

Found in: Antidandruff Shampoos, Antiacne products

Other Names: o-Carboxyphenol, 2-Hydroxybenzoic Acid

Saponins (SAP-ah-nins)

Definition: Saponins are a class of water-soluble, high molecular weight, glycosidal substances that occur naturally in a wide variety of plants.

Class: Biological Products

Function: Surfactants—Cleansing Agent

Found in: Shampoos, Conditioners, Miscellaneous

Other Names: Saponosides

SD Alcohol 40 (SD AL-kuh-hawl)

Definition: SD (specially denatured) alcohol 40 is ethyl alcohol or ethanol, and is the same as that found in alcoholic beverages. Denaturants are added to ethyl alcohol to make it unsuitable for human consumption. Denaturants have an intensely bitter taste that render the alcohol unpalatable. Denatured alcohol is used in hair care products because it is not subject to the consumption tax that must be paid if ethyl alcohol is used as a beverage.

The number after the name indicates the denaturant that has been added. SD alcohol 40 is ethyl alcohol denatured with the addition of t-butyl alcohol and any combination of brucine (alkaloid), brucine sulfate, or quassin.

Class: Alcohols

Function: Solvent, Astringent

Found in: Shampoos, Conditioners, Hairsprays, Setting Lotions, Hair Dyes, Hair Colorants, Permanent Waves, Hair Straighteners, Miscellaneous

Other Names: Denatured Alcohol, Denatured Ethanol, Denatured Ethyl Alcohol

Silica (SIL-ih-kuh)

Definition: Silica is an inorganic oxide that is a naturally occurring mineral. It is used to thicken emulsions and stiffen and improve the setting properties of the hair. It is nontoxic and innocuous.

Class: Inorganics

Function: Thickener and Suspending Agent

Found in: Conditioners, Setting Lotions, Hair Dyes, Hair Colorants, Permanent Waves, Hair Straighteners, Miscellaneous

Other Names: Amorphous Silica, Silicon Dioxide

Silk (SILK)

Definition: Silk is the fibrous protein (mainly fibroin), the biopolymer obtained from the cocoons of the silk worm. Silk protein is structurally similar to hair and regarded as the strongest of the natural fibers.

Class: Proteins

Function: Conditioner

Found in: Shampoos, Conditioners, Hairsprays, Setting Lotions, Hair Dyes, Hair Colorants, Permanent Waves, Hair Straighteners, Miscellaneous

Other Names: Serica

Silk Amino Acids (SILK uh-MEE-noh AS-uds)

Definition: Silk amino acids are a mixture of amino acids that result from the complete hydrolysis of silk protein.

Class: Amino Acids

Function: Conditioners—Moisturizer

Found in: Shampoos, Conditioners, Hairsprays, Setting Lotions, Hair Dyes, Hair Colorants, Permanent Waves, Hair Straighteners, Miscellaneous

Other Names: Silk Protein

Simethicone (si-METH-ih-kown)

Definition: Simethicone is a mixture of dimethicone and silica. It is used in hair care products as an antifoaming and conditioning agent, and imparts a soft, silky feel to the hair.

Class: Siloxanes and Silanes

Function: Conditioners—Moisturizer, Antifoaming Agent

Found in: Shampoos, Conditioners, Setting Lotions, Hair Dyes, Hair Colorants, Permanent Waves, Hair Straighteners, Miscellaneous

Other Names: Silicone Resin, Activated Dimethicone

Sodium Benzoate (SOH-dee-um BEN-zoh-ayt)

Definition: Sodium benzoate is the sodium salt of benzoic acid. It has a long record of safe use as a food preservative and is easily incorporated into hair care products.

Class: Organic Salts

Function: Preservative

Found in: Shampoos, Conditioners, Hairsprays, Setting Lotions, Hair Dyes, Hair Colorants, Permanent Waves, Hair Straighteners, Miscellaneous

Other Names: Benzene Carboxylic Acid, Sodium Salt, Benzoic Acid, Sodium Salt

Sodium Borate (SOH-dee-um BOHR-ayt)

Definition: Sodium borate is an inorganic salt used to adjust the pH of hair care products.

Class: Inorganic Salts

Function: pH Adjuster

Found in: Shampoos, Conditioners, Hairsprays, Setting Lotions, Hair Dyes, Hair Colorants, Permanent Waves, Hair Straighteners, Miscellaneous

Other Names: Borax, Sodium Tetraborate

Sodium Bromate (SOH-dee-um BROH-mayt)

Definition: Sodium bromate is an inorganic salt that is used as an oxidizing agent in hair colorants and permanent waving neutralizers.

Class: Inorganic Salts

Function: Oxidizer

Found in: Permanent Wave Neutralizers, Hair Dyes, Hair Colorants

Other Names: Bromic Acid, Sodium Salt

Sodium Chloride (SOH-dee-um KLOHR-eyed)

Definition: Sodium chloride is an inorganic salt commonly known as table salt. It is used in small quantities to make minor changes in the viscosity of hair care products.

Class: Inorganic Salts

Function: Thickener

Found in: Shampoos, Conditioners, Hairsprays, Setting Lotions, Hair Dyes, Hair Colorants, Permanent Waves, Hair Straighteners, Miscellaneous

Other Names: Table Salt, Common Salt, Rock Salt

Sodium Citrate (SOH-dee-um SY-trayt)

Definition: Sodium citrate is the sodium salt of citric acid.

Class: Organic Salts

Function: pH Adjuster

Found in: Hair Dyes, Hair Colorants

Other Names: Citric Acid Trisodium Salt, Trisodium Citrate

Sodium Cocoamphoacetate (SOH-dee-um KOH-koh-am-foh-ass-uh-tayt)

Definition: Sodium cocoamphoacetate is an amphoteric surfactant.

Class: Alkylamido Alkylamines

Function: Surfactants—Cleansing Agent, Foam Booster, Conditioners—Moisturizer

Found in: Hair Dyes, Hair Colorants

Other Names: Cocoamphoacetate, Cocoamphoglycinate

Sodium Cocoyl Isethionate (SOH-dee-um KOH-coyl eye-SETH-ee-oh-nayt)

Definition: Sodium cocoyl isethionate is the sodium salt of the coconut fatty acid ester of isethionic acid. This mild foaming and cleansing agent was originally developed before the Second World War as a textile detergent, but has found use in shampoos and skin cleansing bars. It is considered milder than sodium lauryl sulfate or sodium laurate.

S

Class: Isethionates
Function: Surfactants—Cleansing Agent
Found in: Shampoos, Skin Cleansing Bars
Other Names: Sodium Cocoyl Ethyl Ester Sulfonate

Sodium Cocoyl Sarcosinate (SOH-dee-um KOH-coyl sar-KOH-sin-ayt)

Definition: Sodium cocoyl sarcosinate is the sodium salt of cocoyl sarcosine. It is a mild foaming and cleansing surfactant that is nonirritating to skin and eyes, and increases the mildness of shampoos.
Class: Sarcosinates and Sarcosine Derivatives
Function: Surfactants—Foam Booster, Cleansing Agent, Conditioner
Found in: Shampoos, Miscellaneous
Other Names: Sodium N-Cocoyl Sarcosinate

Sodium C14-16 Olefin Sulfonate (SOH-dee-um C14-16 OH-lef-in SUL-fuh-nayt)

Definition: Sodium C14-16 olefin sulfonate is a mixture of hydroxyalkane sulfonates and alkene sulfonates derived from C14-16 alpha olefins. They are slightly toxic and irritating, but are milder than lauryl sulfates and similar to lauryl ether sulfates. Sodium C14-16 olefin sulfonate is a high foaming, mild detergent that can be formulated to prepare excellent shampoos.
Class: Sulfonic Acids
Function: Surfactants—Cleansing Agent
Found in: Shampoos, Hair Dyes, Hair Colorants
Other Names: Sodium Tetradecenesulfonate

Sodium C12-15 Pareth Sulfate (SOH-dee-um C12-15 PAYR-eth SUL-fayt)

Definition: Sodium C12-15 pareth sulfate is the sodium salt of a sulfated polyethylene glycol ether of a mixture of synthetic C12-15 fatty alcohols.

Class: Alkyl Ether Sulfates
Function: Surfactants—Cleansing Agent
Found in: Shampoos, Miscellaneous
Other Names: Sodium Pareth-25 Sulfate

Sodium Glutamate (SOH-dee-um GLOO-tuh-mayt)

Definition: Sodium glutamate is the monosodium salt of the L-form of glutamic acid.
Class: Amino Acids
Function: Conditioners—Moisturizer
Found in: Shampoos, Permanent Waving, Straightening, Miscellaneous
Other Names: Monosodium L-Glutamate, Glutamic Acid, Monosodium Salt

Sodium Hyaluronate (SOH-dee-um HI-uh-lur-oh-nayt)

Definition: Sodium hyaluronate is the sodium salt of hyaluronic acid. Although this ingredient is most often used in skin care products, it is also finding use in hair care products.
Class: Biological Polymers and Derivatives
Function: Conditioners—Moisturizer
Found in: Shampoos, Conditioners, Miscellaneous
Other Names: Hyaluronic Acid, Sodium Salt

Sodium Hydroxide (SOH-dee-um hy-DRAHKS-eyed)

S

Definition: Sodium hydroxide is an inorganic alkali commonly known as lye or caustic soda. Many hair care products contain sodium hydroxide, in minor amounts, in order to neutralize acids and adjust the pH of the final product. Although high concentrations of sodium hydroxide are toxic and extremely corrosive, when used in small amounts to adjust the pH of a product, it is neutralized and relatively harmless.

Sodium hydroxide is used, in high concentrations, as the main active ingredient in hydroxide (lye) hair

straighteners. Although hydroxide straighteners are very
effective, caution must be used because of the potential for
excessive damage to both hair and skin.

Class: Inorganic Alkalis

Function: pH Adjuster, Hair Straightening

Found in: Shampoos, Conditioners, Hairsprays, Setting Lotions, Hair Dyes, Hair Colorants, Hair Straighteners, Miscellaneous

Other Names: Caustic Soda, Lye

Sodium Lactate (SOH-dee-um LAK-tayt)

Definition: Sodium lactate is the sodium salt of lactic acid. It
is considered harmless in hair care products and is less
irritating than lactic acid. It is a natural humectant and a
component of the skin, but does not affect its pliability, as
does lactic acid.

Class: Organic Salts

Function: Conditioners—Humectant

Found in: Shampoos, Conditioners, Permanent Waves, Hair
Straighteners, Miscellaneous

Other Names: Sodium Alpha Hydroxypropionate

Sodium Laureth Sulfate (SOH-dee-um LOR-eth SUL-fayt)

Definition: Sodium laureth sulfate is the sodium salt of sulfated ethoxylated lauryl alcohol. Although it is milder than
sodium lauryl sulfate because of the ethoxylation, it is still
considered an irritant. Sodium laureth sulfate is one of the
most common surfactants used in shampoos and other hair
care products.

Class: Alkyl Ether Sulfates

Function: Surfactants—Cleansing Agent, Emulsifying Agent

Found in: Shampoos, Conditioners, Hairsprays, Setting Lotions, Hair Dyes, Hair Colorants, Permanent Waves, Hair
Straighteners, Miscellaneous

Other Names: Dodecyl Sodium Sulfate, Sodium PEG Lauryl
Ether Sulfate

S

Sodium Lauryl Sulfate (SOH-dee-um LOR-il SUL-fayt)

Definition: Sodium lauryl sulfate is an excellent foaming agent, producing rich, thick suds. It is also a powerful detergent and emulsifier for sebum and other oils. Although it is slightly toxic and irritating, it has been used safely for more than 40 years. It became the main surfactant in most shampoos because of its low price, good color, and excellent all-round performance.

But now that milder surfactants with conditioning properties are available, the use of sodium lauryl sulfate has diminished considerably.

Class: Alkyl Sulfates

Function: Surfactants — Cleansing Agent

Found in: Shampoos, Conditioners, Hairsprays, Setting Lotions, Hair Dyes, Hair Colorants, Permanent Waves, Hair Straighteners, Miscellaneous

Other Names: Sodium Dodecyl Sulfate

Sodium Metabisulfite (SOH-dee-um meta-by-SUL-fyt)

Definition: Sodium metabisulfite is an inorganic salt used as an antioxidant and reducing agent.

Class: Inorganic Salts

Function: Antioxidant, Reducing Agent

Found in: Permanent Waves, Hair Straighteners, Hair Dyes, Hair Colorants

Other Names: Sodium Pyrosulfite

S

Sodium Metasilicate (SOH-dee-um meta-SIL-uh-kayt)

Definition: Sodium metasilicate is an inorganic salt used as a chelating agent and corrosion inhibitor.

Class: Inorganic Salts

Function: Chelating Agent

Found in: Hair Dyes, Hair Colorants, Lighteners, Bleaches

Other Names: Disodium Silicate, Sodium Silicon Oxide

Sodium Methyl Cocoyl Taurate (SOH-dee-um METH-ul KOH-coyl TOHR-ayt)

Definition: Sodium methyl cocoyl taurate is the sodium salt of the coconut fatty acid amine of N-methyltaurine. This class of surfactants is considerably milder than sodium lauryl sulfate.

Class: Sulfonic Acids

Function: Surfactants—Cleansing Agent

Found in: Shampoos, Hair Dyes, Hair Colorants, Miscellaneous

Other Names: Amides, Coconut Oil with n-Methyltaurine Sodium Salts

Sodium PCA (SOH-dee-um PCA)

Definition: Sodium PCA is the sodium salt of pyrrolidone carboxylic acid (PCA). This ingredient is a naturally occurring humectant found in skin and a component of the natural moisturizing factor. Sodium PCA has strong water binding properties, more so than propylene glycol, glycerin, or sorbitol. It is a very effective humectant for hair and skin, and is relatively nontoxic and nonirritating.

Class: Amides, Organic Salts, Heterocyclic Compounds

Function: Conditioners—Humectant

Found in: Shampoos, Conditioners, Hairsprays, Aerosol Hairsprays, Setting Lotions, Miscellaneous

Other Names: 2-Pyrrolidone-5-Carboxylic Acid, PCA Soda, Sodium Pyroglutamate

Sodium Perborate (SOH-dee-um pur-BOR-ayt)

Definition: Sodium perborate is an inorganic salt that is used as an oxidizing agent.

Class: Inorganic Salts

Function: Oxidizers

Found in: Permanent Wave Neutralizers, Hair Dyes, Hair Colorants

Other Names: Sodium Peroxoborate

Sodium Persulfate (SOH-dee-um pur-SUL-fayt)

Definition: Sodium persulfate is an inorganic salt that is used as an oxidizing agent. It can cause scalp irritation and is usually found in powdered, off-the-scalp hair lighteners and bleaches.

Class: Inorganic Salts

Function: Oxidizer

Found in: Hair Lighteners, Bleaches

Other Names: Sodium Peroxydisulfate

Sodium Phosphate (SOH-dee-um FAHS-fayt)

Definition: Sodium phosphate is an inorganic salt that is used in small quantities to make minor adjustments in viscosity and to reduce the pH. It is considered to be nontoxic.

Class: Inorganic Salts, Phosphorus Compounds

Function: pH Adjuster, Viscosity Control

Found in: Shampoos, Conditioners, Permanent Waves, Hair Straighteners, Miscellaneous

Other Names: Sodium Biphosphate, Sodium Dihydrogen Phosphate

Sodium Stearate (SOH-dee-um STEER-ayt)

Definition: Sodium stearate is the sodium salt of stearic acid. It is far less irritating than other sodium or potassium soaps. It is considered nontoxic and is used as a food additive. It is added to shampoos and conditioners as a thickener and opacifying agent. It also produces a rich, creamy foam.

Class: Soaps

Function: Thickener, Surfactants—Foam Booster

Found in: Shampoos, Conditioners, Hair Lighteners, Hair Bleaches, Miscellaneous

Other Names: Sodium Octadecanoate

Sodium Sulfate (SOH-dee-um SUL-fayt)

Definition: Sodium sulfate is a naturally occurring inorganic salt that is often found in spring water. It is used in small quantities as a thickener and is considered harmless.

Class: Inorganic Salts
Function: Thickener
Found in: Shampoos, Conditioners, Miscellaneous
Other Names: Glauber's Salt, Disodium Sulfate

Sodium Sulfite (SOH-dee-um SUL-fyt)

Definition: Sodium sulfite is an inorganic salt that acts as an antioxidant, preservative, and reducing agent. It is alkaline in solution, swells hair, and is moderately toxic by ingestion.
Class: Inorganic Salts
Function: Antioxidant, Hair Waving and Straightening—Reducing Agent, Preservative
Found in: Shampoos, Conditioners, Permanent Waves, Hair Straighteners, Hair Dyes, Hair Colorants, Miscellaneous
Other Names: Anhydrous Sodium Sulfite, Sulfurous Acid, Disodium Salt

Sodium Xylenesulfonate (SOH-dee-um zy-leen-SUL-fon-ayt)

Definition: Sodium xylenesulfonate is the sodium salt of ring sulfonated mixed xylene isomers. Although this ingredient increases solvency, it is not considered a surfactant. It is used in small quantities to reduce the viscosity of shampoos and keep the product clear. Sodium xylenesulfonate is used in large quantities in household detergents and although it is considered safe when used in small quantities, it is not considered suitable for hair care products.
Class: Alkyl Aryl Sulfonates
Function: Solvent, Viscosity Control
Found in: Shampoos, Miscellaneous
Other Names: Sodium Dimethylbenzenesulfonate

Soluble Collagen (SAHL-yuh-bul KAHL-uh-jen)

Definition: Soluble collagen is a nonhydrolyzed, native protein derived from the connective tissue of young animals. It consists primarily of tropocallagen, a mixture of the precursors of mature collagen. It is used in hair care products for its moisturizing and film-forming properties. It binds moisture and produces a smooth feeling on skin.

Class: Protein Derivatives

Function: Conditioners — Moisturizer

Found in: Shampoos, Conditioners, Miscellaneous

Other Names: Soluble Animal Collagen, Water Soluble Collagen

Solvent Yellow 172 (SAHL-vent YEL-oh)

Definition: Solvent yellow 172 is a coumarin color used as a hair colorant.

Class: Color Additives

Function: Hair Colorant

Found in: Hair Dyes, Hair Colorants

Other Names: None Available

Sorbic Acid (SOR-bik AS-ud)

Definition: Sorbic acid is an organic acid that occurs naturally in cranberries and mountain ash (the sorbus). It has antimicrobial activity against yeasts and molds, and is used as a food preservative. It is generally recognized as safe.

Class: Carboxylic Acids

Function: Preservative

Found in: Shampoos, Conditioners, Miscellaneous

Other Names: 2,4-Hexadienoic Acid, 2-Propenyl Acrylic Acid

Sorbitan Oleate (SOR-bi-tan OH-lee-ayt)

Definition: Sorbitan oleate is the monoester of oleic acid and hexitol anhydrides derived from sorbitol. It is an emollient used as a superfatting agent and a weak surfactant. It is used as a coemulsifier, emulsion stabilizer, and thickener. It is nontoxic by ingestion.

Class: Sorbitan Derivatives

Function: Surfactants—Emulsifying Agent, Thickener

Found in: Shampoos, Conditioners, Permanent Waves, Hair Straighteners, Miscellaneous

Other Names: Sorbitan Monooleate, Anhydrosorbitol Monooleate

Sorbitol (SOR-bi-tawl)

Definition: Sorbitol is a hexahydric alcohol which occurs naturally in fruits and berries. It is prepared commercially by hydrogenation of D-glucose (dextrose) obtained by hydrolysis of corn starch. It is used in foods as a sweetener and a humectant, and prevents cosmetics from drying out.

Class: Polyols

Function: Conditioners—Humectant

Found in: Shampoos, Conditioners, Hairsprays, Setting Lotions, Hair Dyes, Hair Colorants, Permanent Waves, Hair Straighteners, Miscellaneous

Other Names: D-Glucitol, D-Sorbitol

Squalane (SKWAY-layn)

Definition: Squalane is the saturated branched chain hydrocarbon obtained by hydrogenation of shark liver oil or fish liver oils, and is a by-product of natural vitamin A production. It occurs naturally in human sebum and is nontoxic and nonirritating. It forms an occlusive film on the skin and is used as a moisturizer and conditioner.

Class: Hydrocarbons

Function: Conditioners—Moisturizer

Found in: Shampoos, Conditioners, Hair Straighteners, Miscellaneous

Other Names: Dodecahydrosqualene, Perhydrosqualene

Stearalkonium Chloride (STEER-al-kohn-ee-um KLOHR-eyed)

Definition: Stearalkonium chloride was first used as a textile softener and was the first cationic conditioner used in hair care products. It has excellent conditioning properties and is substantive to the hair. It detangles, improves wet combing, and imparts softness and manageability to hair without making it limp and oily.

Class: Quaternary Ammonium Compounds

Function: Conditioners—Antistatic

Found in: Shampoos, Conditioners, Hairsprays, Setting Lotions, Hair Dyes, Hair Colorants, Permanent Waves, Hair Straighteners, Miscellaneous

Other Names: Stearyl Dimethyl Benzyl Ammonium Chloride

Stearamide DEA (STEER-am-eyed DEA)

Definition: Stearamide DEA is a mixture of ethanolamides of stearic acid. This nonionic surfactant is used as a conditioner, thickener, and foam stabilizer.

Class: Alkanolamides

Function: Surfactants—Foam Booster, Thickener

Found in: Shampoos, Conditioners, Miscellaneous

Other Names: Stearic Acid Diethanolamide

Steareth-10 (STEER-eth 10)

Definition: Steareth-10 is the polyethylene glycol ether of stearyl alcohol. This mild, nonionic surfactant is used as an emulsifier and thickener.

Class: Alkoxylated Alcohols

Function: Surfactants—Emulsifying Agent

Found in: Shampoos, Conditioners, Miscellaneous

Other Names: PEG-10 Stearyl Ether, Polyoxyethylene (10) Stearyl Ether

S

Stearic Acid (STEER-ik AS-ud)

Definition: Stearic acid is both the common name for a commercial blend of hexadecanoic and octadecanoic acids and the trivial name for hexadecanoic acid. It is a product of normal human metabolism. It is nontoxic, nonirritating, and generally recognized as safe. This conditioner is used as an emulsifier when neutralized and in soap form.

Class: Fatty Acids

Function: Surfactants—Emulsifying Agent

Found in: Shampoos, Conditioners, Hairsprays, Setting Lotions, Hair Dyes, Hair Colorants, Permanent Waves, Hair Straighteners, Miscellaneous

Other Names: n-Octadecanoic Acid

Stearyl Alcohol (STEER-ul AL-kuh-hawl)

Definition: Stearyl alcohol is a coemulsifier that is very similar to cetyl alcohol. It is frequently used with cetyl alcohol in a blend known as cetearyl alcohol. Stearyl alcohol is used with surfactants to form creams and lotions, and to stiffen and stabilize hair care products.

Class: Fatty Alcohols, Sulfonic Acids

Function: Surfactants—Emulsifying Agent

Found in: Shampoos, Conditioners, Hairsprays, Setting Lotions, Hair Dyes, Hair Colorants, Permanent Waves, Hair Straighteners, Miscellaneous

Other Names: 1-Octadecanol

Styrene/Acrylates Copolymer (STY-reen/AK-ril-ayts koh-PAHL-uh-mur)

Definition: Styrene/acrylates copolymer is a polymer of styrene and a monomer consisting of acrylic acid, methacrylic acid, or one of their simple esters. It is used in a variety of hair care products as a film former.

Class: Synthetic Polymers

Function: Hair Fixatives, Film Former

Found in: Permanent Waves and Hair Straighteners, Hair Dyes, Hair Colorants

Other Names: 2-Propenoic Acid, Butyl Ester, Polymer with Ethylbenzene

Sucrose (SOO-krohs)

Definition: Sucrose is the disaccharide obtained from sugar cane and sugar beets. It is a humectant and conditioner that is considered harmless.

Class: Carbohydrates, Polyols
Function: Conditioners — Humectant
Found in: Shampoos, Conditioners, Miscellaneous
Other Names: Saccharose, Sugar

Sulfur (SUL-fer)

Definition: Sulfur is a naturally occurring element that is used as an active ingredient (drug) in antidandruff shampoos.
Class: Inorganics
Function: Antidandruff
Found in: Antidandruff Shampoos and Tonics
Other Names: None Available

S

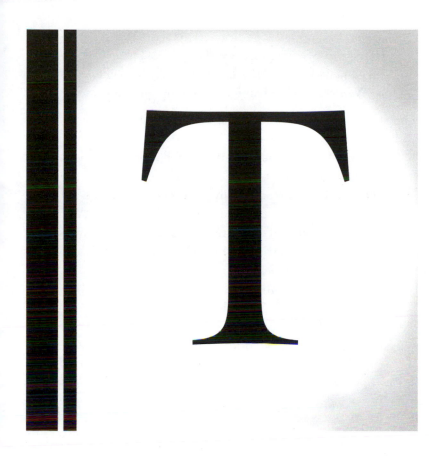

Tallowtrimonium Chloride (tal-oh-TRY-moh-nee-um KLOHR-eyed)

Definition: Tallowtrimonium chloride is a quaternary ammonium salt with alkyl groups derived from tallow. It is a substantive, antistatic conditioner that imparts softness and manageability to hair without giving it a greasy feel. It is slightly toxic and a primary skin and eye irritant.

Class: Quaternary Ammonium Compounds

Function: Conditioners—Antistatic

Found in: Shampoos, Conditioners, Hairsprays, Aerosol Hairsprays, Setting Lotions, Hair Dyes, Hair Colorants, Permanent Waves, Hair Straighteners, Miscellaneous

Other Names: Tallow Trimethyl Ammonium Chloride

TEA-Cocoyl Hydrolyzed Collagen (TEA KOH-koyl HY-droh-lyzed KAHL-uh-jen)

Definition: TEA-cocoyl hydrolyzed collagen is the triethanolamine salt of coconut acid chloride and hydrolyzed collagen. Protein condensates are related to soaps but are milder, and are sometimes used to reduce the irritation of other surfactants. This material has some conditioning and emulsifying properties, but is unlikely to be the main conditioner or emulsifier.

Class: Protein Derivatives

Function: Conditioners—Moisturizer, Surfactants—Cleansing Agent

Found in: Shampoos, Conditioners, Permanent Waves, Hair Straighteners, Miscellaneous

Other Names: Triethanolamine Cocoyl Hydrolyzed Collagen, TEA-Cocoyl Hydrolyzed Protein, TEA-Hydrolyzed Animal Protein

TEA-Lauryl Sulfate (TEA LOR-ul SUL-fayt)

Definition: TEA-lauryl sulfate is the triethanolamine salt of lauryl sulfate where lauryl means C12-14 alcohols. Lauryl alcohol sulfates (ammonium lauryl sulfate and sodium lauryl sulfate) are the standard by which other shampoo surfactants are judged. TEA-lauryl sulfate cleans well, rinses easily, and produces thick, rich foam. Although it is slightly toxic, it can be formulated with other ingredients to reduce irritation. TEA-lauryl sulfate is less popular than ammonium lauryl sulfate, which is cheaper and preferred in acid shampoos.

Class: Alkyl Sulfates

Function: Surfactants—Cleansing Agent

Found in: Shampoos, Hair Dyes, Hair Colorants,
  Miscellaneous
Other Names: Triethanolamine Lauryl Sulfate

Tetrasodium EDTA (tet-rah-SOH-dee-um EDTA)
Definition: Tetrasodium EDTA is a substituted amine similar
  to disodium EDTA but can be slightly more irritating because of its higher pH. Chelating agents are used to stabilize a product and improve its shelf life. They are also used
  in clarifying shampoos.
Class: Alkyl Substituted Amino Acids
Function: Chelating Agent
Found in: Shampoos, Conditioners, Hairsprays, Setting Lotions, Hair Dyes, Hair Colorants, Permanent Waves, Hair
  Straighteners, Miscellaneous
Other Names: Sodium Edetate, Tetrasodium Edetate, Tetrasodium Ethylene Diamine Tetraacetate

Thioglycolic Acid (thy-oh-GLY-kahl-ik AS-ud)
Definition: Thioglycolic acid is a carboxylic acid used in
  permanent waving and hair straightening, and hair
  depilatories.
Class: Thio Compounds, Carboxylic Acids
Function: Hair Waving and Straightening—Reducing Agent,
  Depilatory
Found in: Permanent Waves, Hair Straighteners,
  Depilatories
Other Names: Mercaptoacetic Acid, Thiovanic Acid

Titanium Dioxide (ty-TAYN-ee-um dy-AHK-seyed)
Definition: Titanium dioxide is a naturally occurring
  inorganic oxide, but only synthetic titanium dioxide is
  listed as a color additive in foods, drugs, and cosmetics.
  It is exempt from certification. Titanium dioxide is the
  whitest pigment known and is added to most hair
  care products to intensify their opacity and improve

their color. Titanium dioxide may also be used as an inorganic sunscreen.

Class: Color Additives, Inorganics

Function: Colorant, Sunscreen

Found in: Shampoos, Conditioners, Miscellaneous

Other Names: Pigment White 6, Titanium Oxide

Tocopherol (toh-KAHF-uh-rawl)

Definition: There are four tocopherols of which alpha tocopherol has the highest vitamin E activity. The name has become synonymous with vitamin E. Tocopherols are used as antioxidants, stabilizing essential oils, mineral oils, and vitamin A. Tocopherol is absorbed by the skin. It increases skin elasticity and is used as a moisturizer for dry skin.

Class: Heterocyclic Compounds

Function: Antioxidant, Conditioners—Moisturizer

Found in: Shampoos, Conditioners, Hairsprays, Aerosol Hairsprays, Setting Lotions, Miscellaneous

Other Names: D-Alpha Tocopherol, Mixed Tocopherols, Vitamin E, Natural Vitamin E

Tocopheryl Acetate (toh-KAHF-uh-ril AS-uh-tayt)

Definition: Tocopheryl acetate is the ester of tocopherol and acetic acid. This derivative of tocopherol is used because it is more stable to air, light, and ultraviolet radiation than unesterfied tocopherol. The ester has no antioxidant properties. Tocopheryl acetate is absorbed by the skin and exerts anti-inflammatory effects.

Class: Esters, Heterocyclic Compounds

Function: Conditioners—Moisturizer

Found in: Shampoos, Conditioners, Hairsprays, Aerosol Hairsprays, Setting Lotions, Permanent Waves, Hair Straighteners, Hair Dyes, Hair Colorants, Miscellaneous

Other Names: D-Alpha Tocopheryl Acetate, Vitamin E Acetate

T

Triclocarban (try-KLOH-kar-ban)

Definition: Triclocarban is a substituted carbanilide. This biocide is used as an active ingredient in deodorant soaps and sticks, and antibacterial cleansing products. The long-term effects of exposure to this material are not known.

Class: Amides, Halogen Compounds

Function: Preservative, Cosmetic Biocide, Deodorant

Found in: Deodorant Soaps and Sticks, Antibacterial Cleansing Products

Other Names: TCC, Trichlorocarbanilide

Triclosan (try-KLOH-san)

Definition: Triclosan is a substituted organic ether that is used as a broad-spectrum bactericide in deodorant soaps and sticks, and antibacterial cleansers. It has high percutaneous absorption through intact skin and is not recommended for use in shampoos or hair care products. The long-term effects of exposure to this material are not known.

Class: Ethers, Halogen Compounds, Phenols

Function: Preservative, Cosmetic Biocide, Deodorant

Found in: Deodorant Soaps and Sticks, Antibacterial Cleansing Products

Other Names: None Available

Trideceth-6 (TRY-dek-eth 6)

Definition: Trideceth-6 is a polyethylene glycol ether of tridecyl alcohol with an average value of 6.

Class: Alkoxylated Alcohols

Function: Surfactants—Emulsifying Agent

Found in: Hair Bleaches

Other Names: PEG-6 Tridecyl Ether, Trideth-6

Triethanolamine (try-eth-an-awl-AM-een)

Definition: Triethanolamine is an alkaline substance that is used to adjust the pH of a product or neutralize carboxylic acids. It is prepared by reacting ammonia with ethylene oxide. It is a mild skin and eye irritant. When used to increase pH, it is considered safe for use in products designed for discontinuous, brief use followed by thorough rinsing.

Class: Alkanolamines

Function: pH Adjuster

Found in: Shampoos, Conditioners, Hairsprays, Aerosol Hairsprays, Setting Lotions, Permanent Waves, Hair Straighteners, Hair Dyes, Hair Colorants, Miscellaneous

Other Names: TEA, Trolamine

Trisodium EDTA (try-SOH-dee-um EDTA)

Definition: Trisodium EDTA is a substituted amine that is used as a chelating agent. Many raw ingredients contain trace amounts of iron and other heavy metals. Chelating agents prevent the formation of heavy metal precipitates, the discoloration of a product, and the rancidity of oils or other ingredients.

Class: Amines, Alkyl-Substituted Amino Acids

Function: Chelating Agent

Found in: Shampoos, Conditioners, Hairsprays, Aerosol Hairsprays, Setting Lotions, Hair Dyes, Hair Colorants, Permanent Waves, Hair Straighteners, Miscellaneous

Other Names: Edetate Trisodium, Trisodium Ethylenediamine Tetraacetate

Trisodium HEDTA (try-SOH-dee-um HEDTA)

Definition: Trisodium HEDTA is a substituted amine used as a chelating agent (*see* Trisodium EDTA).

Class: Amines, Alkyl-Substituted Amino Acids

Function: Chelating Agent

Found in: Shampoos, Conditioners, Hairsprays, Aerosol Hairsprays, Setting Lotions, Hair Dyes, Hair Colorants, Permanent Waves, Hair Straighteners, Miscellaneous

Other Names: Trisodium Hydroxyethyl Ethylenediamine Triacetate

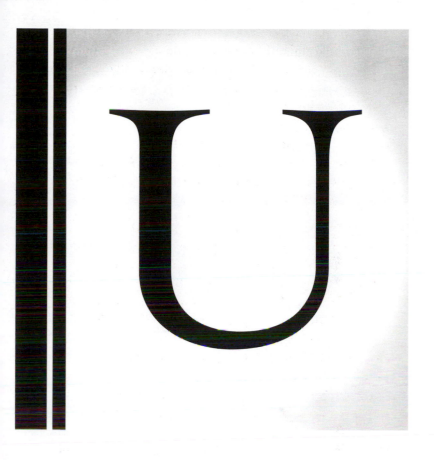

Urea (yoo-REE-uh)

Definition: Urea naturally occurs in urine and other bodily fluids. It is a normal product of human metabolism and is a minor component of the natural moisturizing factor of the skin. It is used in most hair care products as a conditioner. It is used in foods and is considered nontoxic.

Urea has a swelling and softening action on skin and hair (keratin), which explains why it is also used in cuticle removers. Urea may cause irritation when used in high concentrations in topical leave-on creams.

Class: Amides
Function: Conditioners—Humectant
Found in: Shampoos, Conditioners, Setting Lotions, Hair Dyes, Hair Colorants, Hair Bleaches, Permanent Waves, Hair Straighteners, Miscellaneous
Other Names: Carbamide, Urea Perhydrate

U

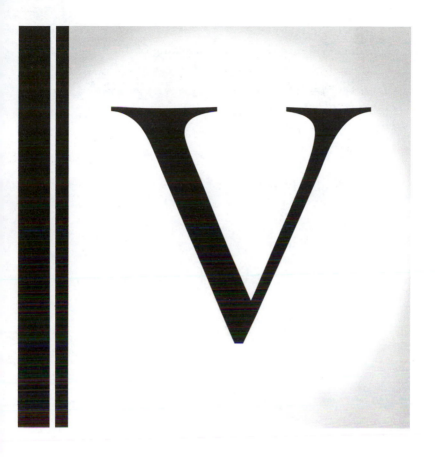

Vegetable Oil (VEJ-tuh-bul OYL)

Definition: Vegetable oil is an expressed oil of vegetable origin consisting primarily of fatty acid triglycerides of fatty acids. The exact oils are not specified. Vegetable oil is used as a superfatting agent and conditioner, and is also a solvent for vitamins.

Class: Fats and Oils

Function: Conditioners—Moisturizer

Found in: Shampoos, Conditioners, Miscellaneous

Other Names: Olus (EU)

Vinegar (VIN-uh-ger)

Definition: Vinegar is a liquid consisting of dilute acetic acid obtained by fermentation.

Class: Biological Products

Function: pH Adjuster

Found in: Shampoos

Other Names: Acetum

Violet 2 (VY-oh-let 2)

Definition: Violet 2 is a batch-certified anthraquinone colorant.

Class: Color Additive

Function: Colorant

Found in: Shampoos, Conditioners, Hairsprays, Aerosol Hairsprays, Setting Lotions, Hair Dyes, Hair Colorants, Hair Bleaches, Miscellaneous

Other Names: D&C Violet #2

VP/VA Copolymer (VP VA KOH-pahl-uh-mur)

Definition: VP/VA copolymer is a synthetic copolymer of vinyl acetate and vinylpyrrolidone monomers.

Class: Synthetic Polymers

Function: Hair Fixative

Found in: Conditioners, Hairsprays, Aerosol Hairsprays, Setting Lotions, Miscellaneous

Other Names: PVP/VA Copolymer, Vinyl AcetateVinylpyrrolidone Copolymer

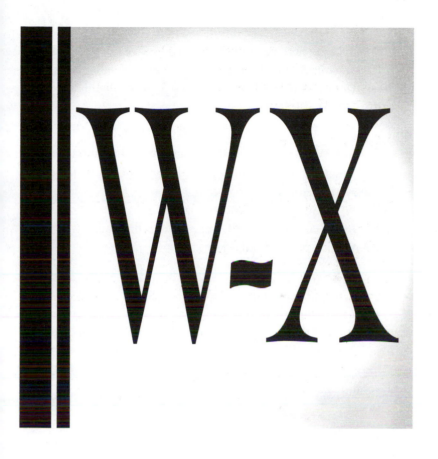

Water (WAW-tur)

Definition: Water is the major ingredient in most hair care products. The exceptions are dry products and hairsprays. Water may contain undesirable trace metal ions that cause discoloration, precipitation, and preservatives to fail. These problems are usually solved by using deionized water that is as pure as commercially possible and by the addition of chelating agents.

Class: Inorganics

Function: Solvent

Found in: Shampoos, Conditioners, Hairsprays, Aerosol Hairsprays, Setting Lotions, Hair Dyes, Hair Colorants, Permanent Waves, Hair Straighteners, Miscellaneous

Other Names: Aqua (EU), Deionized Water, Distilled Water, Purified Water

Wheat Amino Acids (WEET uh-MEE-noh AS-uds)

Definition: Wheat amino acids is a mixture of amino acids that result from the complete hydrolysis of wheat protein.

Class: Amino Acids

Function: Conditioners—Moisturizer

Found in: Shampoos, Conditioners, Miscellaneous

Other Names: None Available

Xanthan Gum (ZAN-than GUM)

Definition: Xanthan gum is a high molecular weight heteropolysaccharide gum produced by pure-culture fermentation of a carbohydrate with *Xanthomonas camestris*. It is a natural polysaccharide produced by biological farming. It is cultured and grown under carefully controlled conditions, then isolated and dried. It is used in hair care products as an emulsion stabilizer and thickener. It also has film-forming and conditioning properties. Xanthan gum is used in foods as a thickener and is considered harmless.

Class: Gums, Hydrophilic Colloids and Derivatives

Function: Thickener, Emulsion Stabilizer

Found in: Shampoos, Conditioners, Setting Lotions, Hair Dyes, Hair Colorants, Hair Bleaches, Miscellaneous

Other Names: Corn Sugar Gum, Xanthan

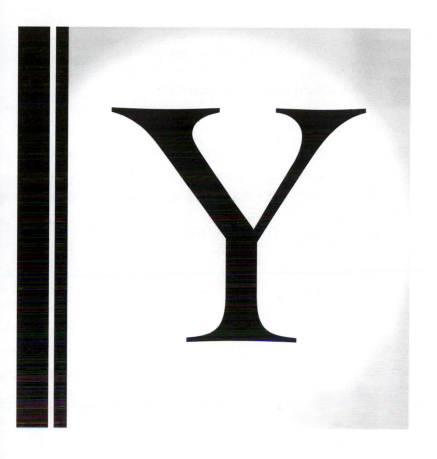

Yeast Extract (YEEST EKS-trakt)

Definition: Yeast extract is prepared from the beer-brewing yeast *Saccharomyces cerevisiae*. It is cultured in a liquid adjusted by the enzymes from barley malt. Yeast contains many components including minerals, vitamins, amino acids, nucleic acids, carbohydrates, lipids, proteins, and enzymes. Extracts are prepared by various means including the use of salt, which is found in the final material. Yeast is used as a conditioner and moisturizer because of its rich content of proteins and saccharides. Autolyzed yeast and hydrolyzed yeast are similar materials.

Class: Biological Products

Function: Conditioners — Moisturizer

Found in: Shampoos, Conditioners, Miscellaneous

Other Names: Faex (EU)

Yellow 6 (YEL-oh 6)

Definition: Yellow 6 is a monoazo color used in hair care products as a colorant.

Class: Color Additives

Function: Colorant

Found in: Shampoos, Conditioners, Miscellaneous

Other Names: FD&C Yellow No. 6

Y

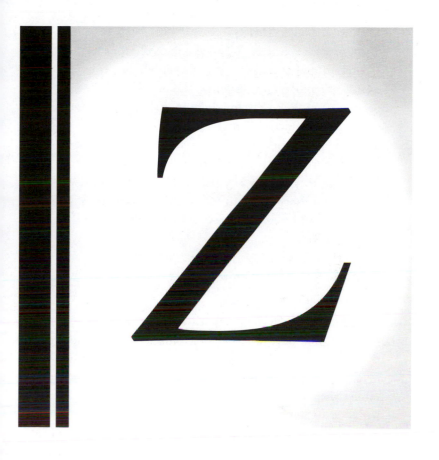

Zinc Acetate (ZINGK AS-uh-tayt)

Definition: Zinc acetate is the zinc salt of acetic acid that is a
well-known astringent, as are many other zinc compounds.
It is often used in aftershave products. It may also have a
slight antiseptic action, but is not considered a preservative. It is considered harmless in small concentrations.

Class: Organic Salts

Function: Astringent

Found in: Shampoos, Conditioners, Miscellaneous

Other Names: Acetic Acid, Zinc Salt

Zinc Oxide (ZINGK AHKS-eyed)

Definition: Zinc oxide is an inorganic oxide that has mild astringent and antiseptic properties, which explains its use in medicinal ointments. It is used in hair care products to whiten cream shampoos and conditioners, and is used in medicated shampoos to achieve a uniform white appearance. It is considered harmless and is a permanently listed color, exempt from batch certification and from any use restrictions. It is also used as a sunscreen agent.

Class: Color Additives

Function: Colorant

Found in: Shampoos, Conditioners, Miscellaneous

Other Names: Pigment White 4, Zinc White

Zinc Pyrithione (ZINGK PUR-ith-ee-own)

Definition: Zinc pyrithione is an aromatic zinc compound that is an extremely effective antidandruff agent. It is a broad-spectrum antimicrobial that is effective against molds, yeasts, and bacteria at low concentrations. It is listed as a Category I (safe and effective) when used as an active ingredient in antidandruff shampoos at concentrations of 1 percent to 2 percent.

Class: Heterocyclic Compounds, Organic Salts, Thio Compounds

Function: Antidandruff, Biocide, Preservative

Found in: Antidandruff Shampoos, Miscellaneous

Other Names: Zinc Pyrithione Suspension

Z

Section IV

Resources

Safety

The U.S. Food and Drug Administration (FDA)
FDA Library
200 C Street, S.W.
Washington, DC 20204
Phone: 202-401-2242 or 202-205-4706
www.fda.gov

**U.S. Department of Labor — Occupational Safety
and Health Administration (OSHA)**
200 Constitution Avenue, N.W.
Washington, DC 20210
Phone: 202-693-1888
www.osha.gov

Research Institute for Fragrance Materials (RIFM)
Two University Plaza
Suite 406
Hackensack, NJ 07601-6209
Phone: 201-488-5527 or 202-293-5800

Cosmetic Ingredient Review (CIR)
1101 17th Street, N
Suite 310
Washington, DC 20036
Phone: 202-331-0651
cirinfo@cir-safety.org
www.cir-safety.org

The Beauty and Barber Supply Institute, Inc. (BBSI)
15825 N 71st Street
Suite 100
Scottsdale, AZ 85254
Phone: 800-468-BBSI
www.bbsi.org.

The Professional Beauty Federation (PBF)
15825 N 71st Street
Scottsdale, AZ 85254
Phone: 703-527-7600, ext. 33
www.probeautyfederation.org

The National Cosmetology Association (NCA)
401 North Michigan Avenue
Chicago, IL 60611
Phone: 312-527-6765
www.beautycity.com

References

Allured Publishing
362 South Schmale Road
Carol Stream, IL 60188
Phone: 630-653-2155
www.Allured.com
www.TheCosmeticSite.com

The Chemistry and Manufacture of Cosmetics (vol. 1–3). Carol
Stream, IL: Allured Publishing.

Schueller, R., & Romanowski, P. (1999). *Beginning Cosmetic
Chemistry.* Carol Stream, IL: Allured Publishing.

Cosmetics and Toiletries Magazine. Carol Stream, IL: Allured
Publishing

Global Cosmetic Industry Magazine
Advanstar Communications, Inc.
131 W. First Street
Duluth, MN 55802-2065
Phone: 800-598-6008
www.advanstar.com

Global Cosmetic Industry Magazine
One Park Avenue
New York, NY 10016
www.globalcosmetic.com
www.cosmeticindex.com

Cosmetic, Toiletry and Fragrance Association, Inc.
1101 17th Street, NW
Suite 300
Washington, DC 20036
Phone: 202-331-1969

CTFA International Cosmetic Ingredient Dictionary and Handbooks, 2002 Edition.

The Society of Cosmetic Chemists (SCC)
120 Wall Street
Suite 2400
New York, NY 10005-4088
Phone: 212-668-1500
www.scconline.org

Brown, K. C., and Pohl, S. (1996). *Monograph Permanent Hair Dyes*. New York: The Society of Cosmetic Chemists.

Rhein, L. D., Peoples, C., & Wolf, B. *Monograph Number 7: Skin, Hair and Nail Structure and Function and Associated Diseases*. New York: The Society of Cosmetic Chemists.

Micelle Press, Inc.
P.O. Box 653
Cranford, NJ 07016

Hunting, A. L. L. (1985). *Encyclopedia of Shampoo Ingredients*. Cranford, NJ: Micelle Press.

Hunting, A. L. L. (1987). *Encyclopedia of Conditioning Rinse Ingredients*. Cranford, NJ: Micelle Press.